BUILDING POSITIVE BEHAVIOR SUPPORT SYSTEMS IN SCHOOLS

BUILDING POSITIVE BEHAVIOR SUPPORT SYSTEMS IN SCHOOLS

FUNCTIONAL BEHAVIORAL ASSESSMENT

DEANNE A. CRONE

ROBERT H. HORNER

THE GUILFORD PRESS

New York   London

© Copyright 2003 The Guilford Press
A Division of Guilford Publications, Inc.
72 Spring Street, New York, NY 10012
www.guilford.com

Figures 2.4, 5.2, and 7.4, and Appendices B, E, and F
© 2003 Deanne A. Crone and Robert H. Horner

Printed in the United States of America

This book is printed on acid-free paper.

Last digit is print number: 9   8   7   6   5   4   3

Library of Congress Cataloging-in-Publication Data

Crone, Deanne A.
    Building positive behavior support systems in schools: functional behavioral assessment / Deanne A. Crone, Robert H. Horner.
        p.   cm.
    Includes bibliographical references and index.
    ISBN 1-57230-818-4 (paper: alk. paper)
1. Behavior modification—United States.   2. Problem children—Education—United States.
I. Horner, Robert H.   II. Title.
LB1060.2.C76 2003
371.39′3—dc21

                                                                                    2002151197

About the Authors

Deanne A. Crone, PhD, is Assistant Professor of School Psychology at the University of Oregon and the Project Director of a federally funded grant to establish and train school-based teams to implement function-based behavior support in elementary and middle schools. Dr. Crone has presented her work on function-based support locally, regionally, and nationally. She has conducted workshops and inservice training for a variety of professionals, including school psychologists, administrators, teachers, and paraprofessionals. In addition, Dr. Crone has written multiple articles on the topic of functional behavioral assessment and positive behavior support.

Robert H. Horner, PhD, is Professor of Special Education at the University of Oregon and Director of Educational Community Supports (ECS), a research unit within the College of Education that focuses on the development and implementation of practices that result in positive, durable, and scientifically validated change in the lives of individuals with disabilities and their families. Dr. Horner's 25-year history of research, grants management, and systems change efforts related to school reform and positive behavior support include helping schools and school administrators develop systems for embedding school-wide systems of positive behavior support.

Acknowledgments

The Department of Special Education and Community Resources at the University of Oregon has formed a group of colleagues, the Functional Assessment Work Group, to discuss and investigate issues related to implementing functional behavioral assessment and positive individual behavior support in general education settings. Collaboration with the Functional Assessment Work Group has been an invaluable resource in the development of this book. We would like to thank the following individuals for their support and contributions: George Sugai, PhD, Anne Todd, MS, Teri Lewis-Palmer, PhD, Tary Tobin, PhD, Rick Albin, PhD, Michelle Shinn, PhD, Shanna Hagan-Burke, PhD , Melissa Bergstrom, MS, Chris Borgmeier, MS, Angelisa Braaksma Fynaardt, PhD, Ben Clarke, PhD, Leanne Hawken, PhD, Joleen Levandowski Doyle, PhD, and Sarah Putra Salentine, BS. Special thanks go to Mike Nelson, PhD and Ted Carr, PhD, for their insightful feedback on early drafts. In addition, we have had the good fortune to work with many talented representatives of local school communities. These individuals have taught us to understand the contextual considerations of implementing functional behavioral assessment and individual behavior support in elementary and middle schools. Our appreciation and recognition goes out to the following individuals: Marilyn Nersesian, Jim Watson, Doris Brown, Kelly Charaun, Susan Taylor-Greene, Doug Kartub, Bruce Stiller, and Kathy White. Finally, we would like to thank the members of the behavior support teams in each of the schools that participated in our school-based functional behavioral assessment training and implementation. Their insights, feedback, and suggestions made a significant contribution to the continued development and improvement of our school-based training model.

Special recognition is due to Melissa Bergstrom, MS, for her significant contributions in developing initial and revised versions of the F-BSP Protocol included in this book.

Preface

WHAT IS THE PURPOSE OF THIS BOOK?

This book is designed as a blueprint for embedding a successful, efficient system of individual behavior support within a school. The goal is to increase your skills in identifying and implementing effective solutions to behavior problems. Part One discusses the contexts and challenges faced in today's schools as a result of serious problem behavior. Part Two illustrates the process of using functional behavioral assessment (FBA) to design and evaluate behavior support plans (BSPs) for three examplary students. Part Three presents the mechanics of what is needed to implement a system of functional behavioral assessment-based behavior support planning (FBA-BSP) within a school.

FOR WHOM IS THIS BOOK WRITTEN?

This book is written for educational personnel (school psychologists, counselors, special educators, teachers, etc.) who lead and serve on behavior support teams. The book also has value for administrators and management teams who have the task of designing behavior support systems and resources.

We have found that schools are most successful in reducing behavior problems when they designate and train a behavior support *team*, instead of relying on only one individual. The success of this team, especially initially, depends on having a member who is skilled in FBA and BSP and who has the ability to efficiently and effectively organize members of the team. This book is written as a guide for the leaders and members of behavior support teams.

WHAT ARE THE INTENDED OUTCOMES OF THIS BOOK?

This book is designed to produce five primary outcomes:

- Describe the professional standards for FBA.
- Provide an efficient and effective model for conducting FBA.
- Define specific procedures for using the results of FBA in the design of behavioral support.
- Define specific procedures for implementing, monitoring, and modifying BSPs.
- Define specific procedures for building the capacity to implement function-based behavior support within a school.

WHAT INVESTMENT IS REQUIRED TO ACCOMPLISH THESE OUTCOMES?

The success of individual behavior support within a school depends on the resources dedicated to ensure sustainability. Sustainability is increased by (1) allocation of sufficient financial and personnel resources, (2) long-term commitment, (3) adequate within-building capacity, and (4) administrative support. Rob Horner, George Sugai, and colleagues (Horner, Sugai, & Todd, 1996) have specified the critical features schools need in order to build a sustainable system of function-based behavior support:

- The school should establish behavior support as one of the top three annual development goals.
- The school should establish a team to address structural change in the school. This team should include an administrator, at least one person with behavior analysis skills, and adequate faculty/staff representation.
- The team should receive training together. Avoid relying on training just one or two people and expecting them to train everyone else. It is important to train 5–10 team members, from each school, together.
- Adequate time and resources should be provided for the team to plan, design, and implement the new procedures.
- The school faculty and staff should be in-serviced on the purpose of the behavior support team and how to gain access to the team's services.
- An evaluation system should be in place to provide regular, accurate information to faculty about the outcomes of the new implementation.

- The new procedures need to produce an outcome valued by all stakeholders while requiring minimal time commitment from teachers.

WHY IS THIS BOOK NEEDED?

Schools face a serious challenge. The incidence and severity of serious behavior problems threaten effective education. On average, 5% of the students within a school account for half or nearly half of all school discipline referrals (Sugai, Sprague, Horner, & Walker, 1999). Students who engage in violent, disruptive, and dangerous behavior compromise the fundamental ability of our schools to educate children, making violent, defiant, disruptive, and dangerous behaviors an issue for all students and all schools.

The bright spot in this picture is that we are now better prepared to prevent and alter patterns of problem behavior than at any time in history (Carr et al., 1999; Gresham, Sugai, Horner, Quinn, & McInerney, 1998; Sugai et al., 2000). A practical and effective technology for responding to problem behaviors, called *functional behavioral assessment* (FBA), has emerged. The technology of FBA can be used to identify the variables supporting problem behaviors and to rearrange the environment to both reduce problem behaviors and build constructive skills (e.g., Ervin, DuPaul, Kern, & Friman, 1998; Lewis & Sugai, 1996). Recently, Carr et al. (1999) reported that in over two-thirds of published studies, interventions using positive behavior support resulted in reducing problem behavior by 80% or more. Of special importance were indications that *interventions were more likely to be effective if they were guided by functional assessment*, conducted in typical settings, conducted by typical personnel, and implemented in a comprehensive manner.

FBA is a powerful and effective technology. It is also a technology that is now *expected* in schools. The 1997 amendments to the Individuals with Disabilities Education Act (IDEA) explicitly recommend that functional assessment information be collected and used to guide behavior support in schools.

Unfortunately, while the results and value of functional assessment are highly acclaimed, there are important limitations to the availability of this technology for school personnel. Functional assessment technology has been characterized by procedures that require very skilled personnel and considerable periods of time. If FBA is to become a basic tool within schools, the efficiency of the procedures (both in terms of who can use them and the amount of time required) must be improved. Responding to this need is a primary focus of this book.

Procedures will be described that were developed in collaboration with school psychologists, teachers, administrators, families, and behavior specialists.

The procedures are designed to fit the needs, skills, and time constraints within typical schools. A major focus of the book will be on the organizational commitments that are essential if FBA and individual behavior support are to be used for real student gains.

WHAT IS FUNCTIONAL BEHAVIORAL ASSESSMENT?

FBA is a method of gathering information about situational events that predict and maintain problem behavior. To obtain this information, the student, his or her teacher(s), and often his or her parents are interviewed about the student's behavior and daily routines. Students also may be observed in the settings in which problem behavior most frequently occurs; in some cases, systematic manipulations of these settings may also be required. The desired outcome of FBA is to (1) obtain an observable and measurable description of the problem behavior; (2) identify the setting events or antecedents that predict when the behavior will and will not occur; and (3) identify the consequences that maintain the problem behavior (O'Neill et al., 1997). This information can be used to generate hypothesis statements that describe the key features of the environment that influence problem behavior.

FBA has several advantages over topological approaches to treatment of serious behavior problems. First, FBA considers individual differences and environmental factors in the development of behavior support plans (O'Neill et al., 1997). Second, the intervention strategies can be directly and logically linked to the problem behavior. FBA links assessment of behavior problems to a choice of intervention strategies by indicating strategies for reducing misbehavior and increasing desired or acceptable alternative behavior (O'Neill et al., 1997). Finally, and most importantly, research suggests that FBA increases treatment effectiveness (DuPaul & Ervin, 1996; Iwata, Dorsey, Slifer, Bauman, & Richman, 1982).

Because children with behavior problems represent a continuum of need, complexity, and risk, the actual process of FBA will not look the same for all students. Children at risk for suspension or alternative school placement due to chronic, severe problem behavior require a more comprehensive assessment than children demonstrating mild, less complex misbehavior.

The model presented in this book recognizes these differences and discusses three different approaches to FBA: simple functional behavioral assessment; full functional behavioral assessment; and functional analysis. Each approach matches the level of staff involvement to the level of need demonstrated by the identified student. Consistent across approaches is an emphasis on problem solving through identification of predictors and consequences of problem behaviors. Each approach requires an observable and measurable definition of the problem behavior. Each approach is discussed in detail in Part One. This three-tiered approach to FBA recognizes the practical realities of limited time and resources in schools. Direct observations of behavior are neither practical nor necessary for every student with problem behavior. For many students with mild problem behaviors, an interview with the teacher (i.e., simple FBA) will suffice to develop a working, testable hypothesis and to design an initial BSP.

Children with more serious or complex problem behavior will require a more extensive assessment, including direct observation in problem settings. Direct observation is an integral part of full FBA and functional analysis.

WHEN IS FUNCTIONAL BEHAVIORAL ASSESSMENT NEEDED?

Schools are required to conduct an FBA for any student with a disability who is at risk for expulsion, alternative school placement, or more than 10 days of suspension. Even though FBA is *required* under limited circumstances, standards of good professional practice dictate a problem-solving approach to managing problem behaviors in the school. Utilizing a function-based approach to problem behavior ensures adherence to standards of professional practice while increasing the school's ability to reduce problem behavior and promote appropriate behavior.

HOW IS THIS BOOK ORGANIZED?

Chapter 1 presents a detailed contextual, historical, and practical discussion of the challenges involved in using FBA within the school system. In Chapter 2, the differences between FBA and traditional approaches to behavioral assessment/intervention are outlined and the consequent implications are discussed. An outline of the process and decision points involved in FBA-BSP is presented. Chapter 3 details the process of conducting an FBA for three examplary students. Observation and interview instruments are introduced. Chapter 4 demonstrates the process of developing an effective, efficient, and relevant BSP for the three examplary students. In Chapter 5, the use of data-based decisions to evaluate and modify the BSP is discussed. Chapter 6 outlines the roles and responsibilities of the individual members of the Behavior Support Team. Chapter 7 addresses critical elements for creating an organized, efficient Behavior Support Team. In Chapter 8, the issue of how to develop within-building capacity (i.e., an array of individuals who have the skills to conduct FBAs and to design, implement, evaluate, and modify BSPs) is outlined. Copies of all relevant forms and instruments are provided in the Appendices.

Contents

**PART ONE. USING FUNCTIONAL BEHAVIORAL ASSESSMENT IN SCHOOLS:
CONTEXTS AND CHALLENGES**

CHAPTER 1 Functional Behavioral Assessment in Schools: 3
The Current Context
Introduction   3
The Context   5
Legislative Demands   5
Availability of Resources and Skills in Schools   6
Maturing Technology   7
Supplementary Section   8

CHAPTER 2 Changing the Way We Think about Assessment   11
and Intervention for Problem Behavior
Introduction   11
Human Behavior Is Functional   11
Human Behavior Is Predictable   12
Human Behavior Is Changeable   13
Assessment   15
Simple Functional Behavioral Assessment   21
Full Functional Behavioral Assessment   23
Functional Analysis   24
Intervention   24

**PART TWO. EMBEDDING FUNCTIONAL BEHAVIORAL ASSESSMENT
WITHIN SCHOOL SYSTEMS: CASE EXAMPLES**

CHAPTER 3 Conducting a Functional Behavioral Assessment   29
Introduction   29
The Assessment Process   30
   *Simple Functional Behavioral Assessment
      (Simple FBA)   35*
   Full Functional Behavioral Assessment (Full FBA)   44
Supplementary Section   54

CHAPTER 4 Designing a Behavior Support Plan   55
Introduction   55
Competing Behaviors   55
Contextual Fit   60
   Example 1   61
   Example 2   61
Individualizing the Behavior Support Plan   62
Documenting a Behavior Support Plan   63
Supplementary Section   68

CHAPTER 5 Evaluating and Modifying the Behavior Support Plan   70
Introduction   70
Rationale   70
Critical Elements   71
   Assessing Changes in Behavior   72
   Documenting the Evaluation Plan   76
   *Assessing Feasibility and Fidelity of Behavior Support
      Plan Implementation   80*
   Assessing Parent, Teacher, and Student Satisfaction   81
Data-Based Decisions   82
Maintenance Plan   84

**PART THREE. USING FUNCTIONAL BEHAVIORAL ASSESSMENT
WITHIN SCHOOL SYSTEMS: QUESTIONS AND CONSIDERATIONS**

CHAPTER 6 Who Will Be Involved in the Behavior Support Team   87
and What Is Needed from Each Person?
Introduction   87
Behavior Support Team Structure   88

Behavior Support Team Membership   91
    School Principal   *91*
    Individual with Competence in Behavioral Assessment
        and Intervention   *92*
    Representative Sample of School Staff   *92*
    Parent   *93*
Behavior Support Team Roles and Responsibilities   93
    Management Roles   *93*
    Performance Roles   *95*

CHAPTER 7 How Do You Get the Behavior Support Team to Work   96
Together as a Team?
Introduction   96
Organizing Structure   97
Organizing Procedure   100

CHAPTER 8 How Do You Generate within-Building Capacity for FBA   110
on the Behavior Support Team?
Introduction   110
    The Challenge   *110*
    The Goal   *111*
Requirements and Commitments   111
    Priorities   *111*
    Resources   *112*
    Continuum of Behavior Support Systems   *114*
A Model for Generating within-Building Capacity   115
    Expected Training Outcomes   *115*
    The Training Model   *116*
Leadership Models   120
    Model 1   *120*
    Model 2   *121*
    Model 3   *121*
Supplementary Section   122

APPENDICES

APPENDIX A Request for Assistance Form   127

APPENDIX B Functional Behavioral Assessment–Behavior Support Plan Protocol   129
(F-BSP Protocol)

APPENDIX C Functional Assessment Checklist for Teachers and Staff (FACTS)   147

APPENDIX D Student-Guided Functional Assessment Interview (Primary)   151

APPENDIX E Assessing Activity Routines Form   153

APPENDIX F Brief Functional Assessment Interview Form   155

APPENDIX G Functional Behavioral Assessment Observation Form   157

APPENDIX H Functional Assessment Observation Form   159

APPENDIX I A Checklist for Assessing the Quality of Behavior Support Planning: 161
Does the Plan (or Planning Process) Have These Features?

References   163

Index   167

BUILDING POSITIVE BEHAVIOR SUPPORT SYSTEMS IN SCHOOLS

PART ONE

Using Functional Behavioral Assessment in Schools: Contexts and Challenges

CHAPTER 1

Functional Behavioral Assessment in Schools: The Current Context

INTRODUCTION

A growing crisis faces students and educators. Student disruption, aggression, and academic failure are a problem in schools nationwide. Students' lack of discipline is viewed in many circles as the biggest problem faced by public schools (National Education Goals Report, 1995), and is a common reason that teachers make requests for assistance from their principal or Student Support Team.

Students with behavior problems are at risk for multiple problems in academic, social, and daily functioning (Loeber & Farrington, 1998). These students are more likely than students without problem behavior to drop out before completing high school; to be suspended, expelled, or placed in alternative school settings; to commit crimes against individuals or the community; to have difficult relationships with their parents and siblings; and to have a higher probability of being arrested (Walker, Colvin, & Ramsey, 1995).

These students not only harm themselves but pose multiple challenges for their administrators, teachers, and fellow classmates. Administrators must spend significant amounts of time responding to teacher, parent, and student needs that accompany problem behavior. Teachers frequently have to interrupt instruction in order to attend to problem behavior. Students with problem behaviors will often require modifications to the curriculum or classroom environment in order to maximize their level of attainment.

Administrators, teachers, parents, and communities often feel overwhelmed and challenged by students with problem behavior. They want to create schools

3

that are places of learning, not places to constantly struggle with misbehavior. Unfortunately, whether because of a lack of training or a lack of resources, many schools do not have the tools or skills to identify and implement effective solutions to behavior problems.

Historically, a common response to problem behavior in schools has been some type of punishment—for example, detention, suspension, or expulsion from school. These reactive approaches serve primarily as short-term solutions that remove the child from the setting. Detention, suspension, and expulsion typically are ineffective at producing long-term reduction of problem behavior, generalization of behavior change, or acquisition of appropriate replacement behaviors (Costenbader & Markson, 1998; Royer, 1995). Clearly, schools need something more than a reactive approach to behavior management.

Multiple behavioral interventions other than detention and suspension can successfully reduce problem behavior in children (Dwyer, Leeming, Cobern, Porter, & Bryan, 1993; Gresham, Gansle, Noell, Cohen, & Rosenblum, 1993). In fact, schools currently have access to some of the most effective strategies for behavior support ever available. *The challenge is to embed these strategies in the complex and demanding culture of our schools.*

One of the most difficult challenges in designing effective interventions for children with problem behavior is the highly variable, individual response to intervention. Strategies that work for one child may have no impact on the behavior of another child with similar behavior. Even so, behavior intervention plans are often built in response to the type of behavior (e.g., fighting, stealing, vandalism, profanity), rather than in response to the individual characteristics of the student or setting.

To plan a successful intervention, the interventionist should consider more than the problem behaviors and a menu of intervention options: *What typically triggers the problem behavior? What reward does the student obtain by engaging in the problem behavior?* Given the variety of interventions that could be applied, teachers and school staff need a means for deciding which intervention or combination of interventions will be most effective for an individual student within a specific school setting. Functional behavioral assessment (FBA), when linked to the development of behavior support plans (BSPs), is an effective and efficient tool for addressing this need. (Note: This book is not intended as a primer on FBA or behavior management. There are a number of excellent resources on both these topics, many of which are listed in the Supplementary Section to this chapter. We assume that the reader of this book has knowledge and experience in functional behavioral assessment-based behavior support planning [FBA-BSP], but requires practical assistance in effectively and efficiently embedding FBA-BSP into the school infrastructure.)

Although federal laws require schools to use FBA in certain circumstances, many school personnel are unaware of the technology, let alone competent to use it. Ironically, at the same time, there have been exciting, recent research advances in the technology of FBA-BSP that have direct relevance for addressing violent and disruptive behavior in schools (e.g., Dunlap, White, Vera, Wilson, & Panacek, 1996; Mayer, 1995) *The immediate challenge is to transform these research advances into an accessible technology that school psychologists, teachers, and administrators can apply in typical school settings.*

THE CONTEXT

Legislative Demands

Based on compelling evidence documenting its effectiveness, FBA has become expected professional practice mandated by state regulations in California, Oregon, Washington, Minnesota, New York, and Florida (Turnbull, Rainbolt, & Buchele-Ash, 1997; Wilcox, Turnbull, & Turnbull, 1999–2000). In some cases, FBA is required by law. In 1997, the U.S. Congress reauthorized the Individuals with Disabilities Education Act (IDEA). Amendments to the IDEA (1997) included a recommendation that schools use FBA procedures to develop support strategies for children with disabilities who display severe behavior problems. A functional assessment of behavior is *required* before a school suspends (for more than 10 days) or expels a student with a disability. The following excerpts from the reauthorization of IDEA clarify the role of the school and the Individualized Education Plan (IEP) team in addressing the behavioral problems of children with disabilities:

- The IEP Team shall in the case of a child whose behavior impedes his or her learning or that of others, consider, when appropriate, strategies, including positive behavioral interventions, strategies, and supports to address that behavior (614[d][3][B][i]);
- Either before or not later than 10 days after taking a disciplinary action (change in the placement of a child with a disability to an appropriate interim alternative educational setting, another setting, or suspension, for not more than 10 school days), if the local educational agency did not conduct a functional behavioral assessment and implement a behavioral intervention plan to address that behavior; or if the child already has a behavioral intervention plan, the IEP Team shall review the plan and modify it, as necessary, to address the behavior (615[k][1][B]); and
- Each State improvement plan shall describe . . . how the State will address the identified needs for in-service and pre-service preparation to ensure that all personnel who work with children with disabilities (including both professional and paraprofessional personnel who provide special ed-

ucation, general education, related services, or early intervention services) have the skills and knowledge necessary to meet the needs of children with disabilities (653[c][3][D][vi]).

As members of IEP teams, these educators play an ever-increasing role in collaboratively developing comprehensive management and instructional plans for students with disabilities. For many educators, the use of FBA to design individualized behavior support strategies is a new role requiring new skills. Many school personnel are finding themselves under legislative pressure to deliver services for which they do not have the necessary knowledge, training, or resources.

AVAILABILITY OF RESOURCES AND SKILLS IN SCHOOLS

For many educators, using a function-based approach to explain problem behavior will require a shift in their theoretical perspective. School personnel may view problem behavior primarily as the result of poor parenting, developmental/mental illness (e.g., autism, Attention-Deficit/Hyperactivity Disorder), or personality traits. In other words, they see problem behavior as more a result of within-person pathology than as a result of environmental events or routines. While such characteristics certainly may contribute to problem behavior, a within-child focus is less useful in identifying environmental variables that can be altered within the school or classroom to improve the student's behavior. Learning to develop BSPs based on FBA information requires more than just learning a new skill; *it requires learning and accepting a new conceptualization of problem behavior.*

Schools differ in the extent to which they are prepared to develop and implement a system of function-based behavior support. Some schools employ a school psychologist or an outside behavior consultant. Other schools assign several staff members to serve as a Behavior Support Team for students with serious behavior problems. The extent to which these individuals or teams are qualified and effective will vary tremendously. Many schools have not identified any system for conducting FBAs and for developing individualized BSPs. Instead, they may rely on detention, suspension, special education placement, or outside referral to cope with the problem behaviors in their school. Part Three addresses how the school psychologist or the leader of the Behavior Support Team can help build a sustainable system of function-based behavior support within a school by developing an efficient organizational structure, organizational procedures, and skill fluency among team members.

Maturing Technology

FBA procedures have been in use for more than 25 years (Carr, 1977). However, only recently has FBA been used or recommended for use in regular education settings (IDEA, 1997).

Changing Population

Historically, FBA was most often applied in outpatient or clinical settings for developmentally delayed adults with serious behavior problems (Carr et al., 1999). Conducting an FBA has typically been a time-intensive procedure that required a highly trained behavior analyst. IDEA (1997) now recommends using members of the Individualized Education Plan (IEP) team to conduct FBA of problem behavior for a student with a disability in regular school settings. Some researchers have criticized the amendments to IDEA (1997), counseling that the new legislative policy mandates the use of FBA in contexts that are too far removed from its empirically documented uses (Nelson, Roberts, Mather, & Rutherford, 1999). Although this is a valid point, it is not feasible to delay the implementation of FBA in general education settings. The amendments to IDEA (1997) have established FBA-BSP as a necessary part of standard required practice. At this point, the challenge is to provide adequate training and support to schools to include FBA-BSP, while conducting research to test and improve the use of FBA-BSP in general education settings.

Furthermore, initial investigations suggest that FBA can be feasibly implemented in general education settings with students with mild or no disabilities, and that BSPs based on FBA are effective in reducing problem behavior and increasing appropriate behavior for these students (e.g., Broussard & Northrup, 1995; Dunlap ct al., 1996; Eccles & Pitchford, 1997; Reed, Thomas, Sprague, & Horner, 1997; Sugai, Bullis, & Cumblad, 1997).

Increased Efficiency of Procedures

The authors and their colleagues have developed time-efficient interview and observation tools to collect information on problems behaviors and their antecedents and consequences. Some of these tools will be presented and discussed in Part Three of this manual. Blank copies of all these forms are available in the Appendices.

The process of FBA can be expedited through accountability, good organization, and close attention to time management. Simple procedures such as regularly scheduled meetings, time-limited agendas, detailed action plans, and centralized record keeping can significantly improve time usage. These and other procedures for making the best use of time are discussed in detail throughout this book.

The efficiency of function-based behavior support can be further improved by recognizing that the intensity of the assessment process can vary depending on the complexity and severity of the problem behavior. Not every child who is referred for problem behavior requires a *full* FBA.

For many children, the problem behavior can be adequately assessed by conducting a simple FBA. The simple FBA relies on a brief teacher interview to define the problem behavior and identify the antecedents and consequences of that problem behavior. An effective BSP can be built on this limited information. The simple FBA would be appropriately applied in situations where (1) the problem behavior is not severe or complex; (2) the team has a high level of confidence that the relevant antecedents, consequences, and functions have been identified through the teacher interview; and (3) the child is not in danger of suspension, expulsion, or alternative school placement.

Children with complex, severe, or at-risk problem behavior will require a full FBA. A full FBA is also appropriate if a child's behavior is not severe, but the team lacks confidence in the testable hypothesis generated from the initial teacher interview. A full FBA includes direct observations of the student in at least two settings. Interviews with additional teachers, the parents, and the child and a review of the child's school records are often included as well.

A small percentage of children may require a functional analysis of behavior to accurately assess and effectively intervene in the problem behavior. Functional analysis involves experimental manipulation of antecedents and consequences to increase the precision and accuracy of the assessment. Functional analyses must be carried out by an individual with experience in applied behavior analysis.

Because of limited existing resources, schools will require a comprehensive model of FBA that is efficient, effective, and inclusive, yet can be adapted to fit the different challenges these children represent. This book will explain a three-tiered model (simple FBA, full FBA, and functional analysis) and delineate a decision-making process to distinguish between the three options.

SUPPLEMENTARY SECTION

Conducting Functional Assessments

- O'Neill, R. E., Horner, R. H., Albin, R. W., Sprague, J. R., Storey, K., & Newton, J. S. (1997). *Functional assessment and program development for problem behavior: A practical handbook*. (2nd ed.). Pacific Grove, CA: Brooks/Cole.

Tools for Conducting Functional Assessment Interviews

- Assessing Activity Routines Form (see Appendix E).
- Brief Functional Assessment Interview Form (see Appendix F).
- Function-based-Behavior Support Plan Protocol (see Appendix B).
- Functional Assessment Checklist for Teachers and Staff (see Appendix C).
- Functional Assessment Interview, in R. E. O'Neill, R. H. Horner, R. W. Albin, J. R. Sprague, K. Story, & J. S. Newton (1997), *Functional assessment and program development for problem behavior: A practical handbook.* (2nd ed.). Pacific Grove, CA: Brooks/Cole.
- Student-Guided Functional Assessment Interview (see Appendix D).

Tools for Conducting Functional Assessment Observations

- Functional Assessment Observation Form in R. E. O'Neill, R. H. Horner, R. W. Albin, J. R. Sprague, K. Story, & J. S. Newton (1997), *Functional assessment and program development for problem behavior: A practical handbook.* (2nd ed.). Pacific Grove, CA: Brooks/Cole. (see Appendix H).
- Functional Behavioral Assessment Observation Form, in G. Sugai & J. Tindal (1993), *Effective school consultation.* Pacific Grove, CA: Brooks/Cole. (see Appendix G).

Tools for Developing Behavior Support Plans

- Function-based-Behavior Support Plan Protocol (F-BSP Protocol) (see Appendix B).
- A Checklist for Assessing the Quality of Behavior Support Planning. Adapted from Horner, R. H., Sugai, G., Todd, A. W., & Lewis-Palmer, T. (1999–2000). Elements of behavior support plans: A technical brief. *Exceptionality, 8,* 205–216 (see Appendix I).

Behavior Management

- Colvin, G. (1992). *Managing acting-out behavior: A staff development program.* Eugene, OR: Behavior Associates (distributed by Sopris West, Longmont, CO).
- Colvin, G., & Sugai, G. (1989). *Managing escalating behavior* (2nd ed.). Eugene, OR: Behavior Associates.
- Koegel, L. K., Koegel, R. L., & Dunlap, G. (Eds.). (1996). *Positive behavioral support: Including people with difficult behavior in the community.* Baltimore: Brookes.
- Nelson, C. M., & Rutherford, R. B., Jr. (1988). Behavioral interventions with behaviorally disordered students. In M. C. Wang, M. C. Reynolds, & H. J. Walberg (Eds.), *Handbook of special education: Research and practice* (Vol. 2, pp. 125–153). Oxford, UK: Pergamon Press.
- Repp, A. C., & Horner, R. H. (Eds.). (1999). *Functional analysis of problem behavior: From effective assessment to effective support.* Belmont, CA : Wadsworth.

Interventions for Schoolwide, Classroom, or Non-Classroom-Specific Settings

- Cangelosi, J. S. (1988). *Classroom management strategies: Gaining and maintaining students' cooperation.* White Plains, NY: Longman.
- Charles, C. M. (1989). *Building classroom discipline: From models to practice* (3rd ed.). White Plains, NY: Longman.
- Kartub, D. T., Taylor-Greene, S., March, R. E., & Horner, R. H. (2000). Reducing hallway noise: A systems approach. *Journal of Positive Behavioral Interventions, 2*(3), 179–182.
- Lewis, T. J. & Garrison-Harrell, L. (1999). Effective behavior support: Designing setting-specific interventions. *Effective School Practices, 17*, No. 4 (pp. 38–46). Eugene, OR: Association for Direct Instruction.
- Sprick, R. S., & Howard, L. M. (1995–1997). *The teacher's encyclopedia of behavior management.* Longmont, CO: Sopris West.
- Sprick, R., Sprick, M., & Garrison, M. (1993). *Interventions: Collaborative planning for students at risk.* Longmont, CO: Sopris West.
- Taylor-Greene, S., Brown, D., Nelson, L., Longton, J., Gassman, T., Cohen, J., Swartz, J., Horner, R. H., Sugai, G., & Hall, S. (1997). School-wide behavioral support: Starting the year off right. *Journal of Behavioral Education, 7*(1), 99–112.

Crisis Plans

- Fairchild, T. N. (1997). School-based helpers' role in crisis intervention. In T. N. Fairchild (Ed.), *Crisis intervention strategies for school-based helpers* (pp. 3–19). Springfield, IL: Charles C. Thomas.
- Parks, A. L., & Fodor-Davis, J. (1997). Managing violent and disruptive students. In T. N. Fairchild (Ed.), *Crisis intervention strategies for school-based helpers* (pp. 245–277). Springfield, IL: Charles C Thomas.
- Sprick, R., Sprick, M., & Garrison, M. (1993). *Interventions: Collaborative planning for students at risk.* Longmont, CO: Sopris West.

CHAPTER 2

Changing the Way We Think about Assessment and Intervention for Problem Behavior

INTRODUCTION

In a function-based approach, effective solutions to problem behaviors focus on environmental events (not within-person pathologies) that trigger and maintain problem behavior. For many school personnel, this emphasis on changing the student's environment rather than "fixing the person" represents a dramatic shift in philosophy. Therefore, before implementing function-based behavior support, it is important to appreciate three assumptions that serve as a foundation for FBA systems: (1) human behavior is functional, (2) human behavior is predictable, and (3) human behavior is changeable.

Human Behavior Is Functional

The primary principle of function-based behavior support is that people act the way they do for a reason. That is, most behavior is functional: it serves a purpose. The function of the behavior may be to obtain something the person wants, to generate adult or peer attention, or to escape from an aversive situation or person. The results or consequences of a behavior affect the future occurrence of that behavior. As intelligent, discerning individuals, students begin to recognize that some strategies are more effective than others at producing the outcomes they desire. Students will use effective strategies more often than ineffective strategies. For example, a student who wants to be part of the cheerleading squad learns that practicing the routines and consistently attending tryouts on time is more effective than complaining that tryouts are unfairly biased toward the "popular" girls.

Ironically, students sometimes learn that *problem behavior* can be more efficient than appropriate behavior in producing desired outcomes. This may be true in cases when a student gets out of a difficult assignment by having a temper tantrum in class or when a student becomes the center of attention for his peers by swearing at a teacher. Much to the dismay of the school staff, these students recognize that inappropriate behavior can be an effective strategy for obtaining what they want. As a result, their problem behavior continues or intensifies. For example, consider the following cases:

> James is a seventh-grade student with difficulties in oral reading. In social studies class, each student is expected to take a turn reading part of the chapter out loud. When it is James's turn, he responds by having a tantrum: he throws his books on the floor and swears at his teacher. His teacher responds by sending him to the vice-principal's office. This problem behavior continues and worsens.

> Michael, a second-grade student, pushes the other children in line when he is told to stand at the end of the line. When the teacher lets him hold the door, he stops pushing. This happens every time the students line up for lunch. The problem behavior continues on a daily basis.

> Lisa is a fifth-grade student who loves to be the center of attention. She frequently makes loud inappropriate jokes in class that cause her classmates to laugh. This behavior continues even though the teacher interrupts each incident by giving Lisa a long lecture about appropriate fifth-grade behavior.

Despite the disruption and frustration caused by each of these students, their behaviors are understandable within the given context. Each student is achieving his/her desired outcome (escaping embarrassment, obtaining a privilege, or receiving peer attention) by engaging in inappropriate, not appropriate behavior. The inappropriate behavior is serving a function for each student.

Human Behavior Is Predictable

Human behavior does not occur in a vacuum. Environmental conditions can set up, set off, or maintain problem behavior. Take, for example, the case of James. James is embarrassed by his poor oral reading skills. Although his teacher is aware of his reading difficulties, she is mystified by his problem behavior. She views his behavior as unpredictable and does not understand why he is undeterred by her numerous referrals to the vice-principal's office. After closer analysis, the Behavior Support Team notes two important contributors to James's behavior. First, his problem behavior occurs most frequently in situations when he is expected to read out loud in a large-group setting. This environmental condition serves as a *predictor*, or *antecedent*, for James's problem behavior. Second, when James is sent to the office for problem behavior, he escapes the embarrassment of stumbling through a reading passage in front of his friends. Like many preadolescents, James would rather have his friends believe that he is a troublemaker than have them find out that he is a poor reader. In this case, the *consequence* of being sent to the office is rewarding to James. In fact, James has learned that if he wants to get out of reading in front of the class, he *must* have a tantrum. By looking for the antecedents and consequences that set up and maintain James's tantrums, his problem behavior becomes very predictable.

Human Behavior Is Changeable

Not only can we predict behavior, but we can change it as well. Understanding the functions, predictors, and consequences of problem behavior helps us to pinpoint and script the appropriate behavioral interventions. A *functional* assessment of behavior switches the focus from "treatment of within-child pathology" to "design of effective environmental routines." The Behavior Support Team learns to analyze problematic routines (e.g., oral reading during James's social studies class) and decide on how to make feasible, practical changes to these routines to promote the behavioral success of the identified student.

A behavioral intervention has two primary goals: to *reduce problem behavior* and *to increase appropriate behavior*. Meeting these goals will often require comprehensive changes in the student's routine, repertoire of skills, or interactions with adults. There are at least three means to meet these goals:

1. *Make the problem behavior irrelevant.* Decrease or eliminate the need to engage in the behavior.
2. *Make the problem behavior inefficient.* Provide the child with a replacement behavior that serves the same function as the inappropriate behavior.
3. *Make the problem behavior ineffective.* Do not allow the child to obtain what he or she wants through inappropriate behavior.

Make the Problem Behavior Irrelevant

Altering a problematic routine by altering its predictors often makes the problem behavior irrelevant. For example, Susan was referred for extreme distractibility during reading and math instruction. A FBA of Susan's behavior and her environmental routines yielded two important findings: (1) math and reading instruction took place during the morning; (2) Susan was often sent to school without breakfast. The Behavior Support Team concluded that Susan's distractibility was a direct result of her hunger. They altered her environmental routine by sending Susan to the school cafeteria every morning for breakfast. Once Susan had eaten in the morning, her distractibility in math and reading was eliminated. In other words, the problem behavior was made *irrelevant* by an inexpensive, practical change in the student's routine. Often, it can be less time- and labor-intensive to change a problem behavior by changing its predictors than by changing the consequences of the behavior (Luiselli & Cameron, 1998).

Make the Problem Behavior Inefficient

Teachers and educators usually do not consider the *function* of problem behavior to be inappropriate or offensive. Teachers understand that students want to solicit attention, escape aversive situations, and receive tangible rewards and privileges. Rather, it is the *means* that the student uses to achieve the end (the function) that is problematic. A critical component of an effective behavioral intervention is teaching the child an appropriate replacement behavior that serves the same function as the inappropriate behavior. If a child can achieve his desired end without damaging his relations with peers or teachers, the problem behavior becomes less efficient than the appropriate behavior. The child will begin to use the replacement behavior more frequently.

In a previous example, James would have a temper tantrum in order to get out of an embarrassing situation. The Behavior Support Team must teach James an alternate behavior that serves the same function as the tantrum, without resulting in detention or in-school suspension. The team could teach James to ask for a 2-minute break when he is feeling overwhelmed by the assignment. Alternatively, the team could ask the teacher to give James silent reading assignments matched to his reading ability to replace the oral reading tasks. Both of these options serve the same function as James's tantrum: to provide him with relief from the embarrassment of a publicly challenging academic situation. The alternative behaviors, however, are much more acceptable to James's teacher than his temper tantrums. The problem behavior is rendered *inefficient*. James can now escape his embarrassment without creating a negative situation for himself and his teacher.

Make the Problem Behavior Ineffective

From the student's point of view, problem behavior works. It may get her out of a difficult situation or it may help her obtain something she wants. Imagine the preschool child who wants to eat a cookie before lunchtime. Initially, the teacher says no. The child begins to whine. The teacher holds her ground and sends the child to time-out for whining. The child gets louder and more adamant. Finally, the teacher gives in and gives the child the cookie. Rather than learning that she will get in trouble for whining, the child learns that she just needs to whine louder and longer to get what she wants! In order to make problem behavior in-effective, the Behavior Support Team must identify the consequences that main-tain the problem behavior. The maintaining consequences must then be elimi-nated. By eliminating the maintaining consequences (e.g., giving in to whining), the child learns that the problem behavior is not an *effective* strategy for obtain-ing the desired outcome.

ASSESSMENT

• *How do I know if the problem behavior is a result of an individual problem or a systemswide problem?* Within this book, we present a model for developing, embedding, and maintaining a system of function-based behavior support within a school. We will focus on building a model that meets the full range of behavioral challenges presented in a school.

The first challenge is to recognize that there are several systems within a school where behavioral concerns are an issue: schoolwide, classroom, common non-classroom specific areas (e.g., the cafeteria, hallways, the playground, etc.), and individual students (see Figure 2.1). Each system exists within every school. Each system overlaps and impacts the others. Each system is a setting that can set off and maintain problem behaviors or that can be redesigned to reduce problem behaviors (Todd, Horner, Sugai, & Colvin, 1999).

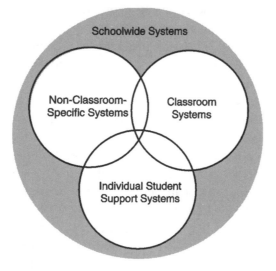

FIGURE 2.1. Behavioral systems within every school. From Horner, Sugai, Todd, & Lewis- Palmer (1999). Copyright 1999–2000 Lawrence Erlbaum Associates. Reproduced by permission of Law-rence Erlbaum Associates.

Sugai and colleagues (1999) have developed a method for pinpointing within a school those systems that are in need of intervention. This method is based on examining patterns in school discipline referral records. All the discipline referrals in the building are entered into an easy-to-use database on a daily basis. Simple bar graphs can be generated from the database to illustrate different patterns in the discipline referrals. The authors of this book recommend a Web-based system called the School-Wide Information System (SWIS) for recording and analyzing discipline referral data. Information about SWIS is available online at *www.swis.org*. Contact information for obtaining SWIS is listed in the Supplementary Section of this chapter.

If a large proportion of the student body (i.e., more than 35%) has had at least one office referral within a school year, the school has a schoolwide problem in delivering effective behavior support. A problem at the schoolwide level would dictate an intervention at the schoolwide level. One solution would be to identify four or five basic behavioral expectations and then teach, model, and practice these behavioral expectations with all the students in the school (Taylor-Greene et al., 1997).

If a disproportionate number of referrals originate in one or two classrooms, only those particular classrooms may be in need of behavioral intervention. Similarly, if the majority of the problems seem to originate in just one or two settings, such as on the playground or in the cafeteria, the problem is at the level of common areas. Finally, if a small percentage of students are responsible for a large percentage of referrals, then the problem is at the individual systems or targeted-group level. *These individuals are identified as the students who can benefit from function-based behavior support.*

Figures 2.2 and 2.3 demonstrate how this methodology is used. Figure 2.2 illustrates the number of discipline referrals for one school, by location. For this school, the majority of the behavior problems are occurring in the classroom, commons, and playground. Thus, the Behavior Support Team would conclude that their efforts should be concentrated on improving behavior in these areas.

Figure 2.3 illustrates the number of referrals that each student in the database has received. (Students who never receive a referral are not entered into the database.) In this school less than 35% of the total school population has received one or more referrals. The Behavior Support Team can logically conclude that the universal interventions they have in place are effective in reducing problem behavior for the majority of students. This Behavior Support Team can thus turn its attention to individual students. The 1–7% of students producing the most referrals are probably the best candidates for function-based behavior support. If a school is using a database system similar to SWIS, the team will be able to generate a report for an individual student that provides detailed information on each of that student's referrals listed in the database.

Schools may experience problems in one or more of the identified systems.

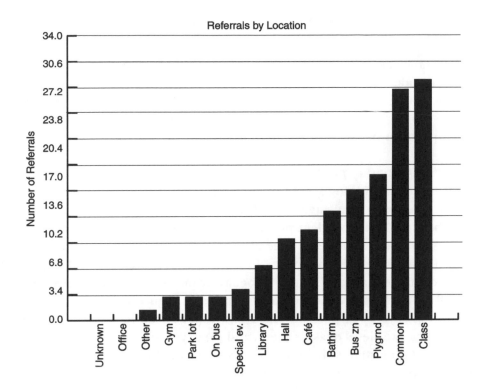

FIGURE 2.2. Discipline referrals by location.

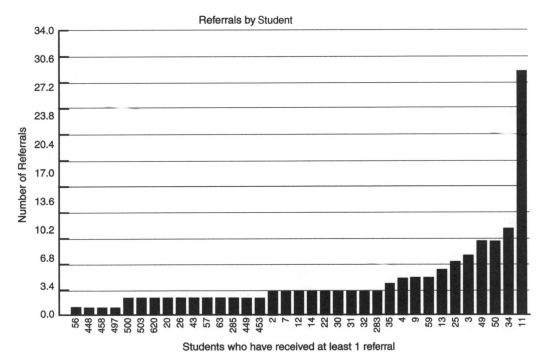

FIGURE 2.3. Discipline referrals by student.

Techniques for assessing and managing problem behaviors within each system have been widely documented. (The Supplementary Sections in Chapters 1 and 8 provide a list of references for interventions at the schoolwide, classroom, and non-classroom-specific levels). This book will demonstrate how to assess and manage problem behavior at the *individual student system* level.

• *What percent of problem behavior occurs at the individual student system level?* After examining school discipline records, school officials may be surprised to find that, on average, half of school discipline referrals are accounted for by about 5% of the student population (Sugai et al., 1999). On the positive side, these statistics indicate that the majority of a school's enrollment is not engaging in serious problem behaviors. In fact, 80–85% of students will respond favorably to simple, universally applied behavior management strategies (Sugai et al., 1999). The Behavior Continuum Triangle in Figure 2.4 provides a breakdown of the severity of problem behaviors experienced in a school by (1) system, (2) suggested level of assessment, and (3) suggested level of intervention.

Figure 2.4 illustrates that the resources allocated to assessing the problem and designing an intervention should be matched proportionally to the level and intensity of the problem. For example, if an analysis of discipline referral patterns indicates that recurring behavior problems exist on the playground, assessment should be directed toward determining the features of the playground that increase the likelihood that problems will occur. *Are there areas of the playground that are hidden from adult view? Are there too many children to share limited equipment? Are there too few supervisors to ensure the safety of the children on the playground?* Once the assessment has determined the dysfunctional features of the non-classroom-specific system, interventions should be directed at changing those features.

• *What percentage of referrals at the individual student system level will require simple functional behavioral assessment, full functional behavioral assessment, or functional analysis?* The Behavior Support Team will be concerned with those 1–15% of students whose problem behavior places them at the top of the Behavioral Continuum Triangle (see Figure 2.4). These students can be further differentiated.

Discipline referrals may indicate that some students are at risk for developing patterns of serious problem behavior, but the problem has not yet become serious, dangerous, or chronic. These students may benefit from a targeted-group intervention that can be individualized with a simple FBA. For example, a school may institute a "Check-in/Check-out" system. In this system, a group of students at risk for developing serious problem behavior is identified. Each student is given a behavior card that lists up to five behavioral goals. At the beginning of the day each student "checks in" with the same educational assistant to

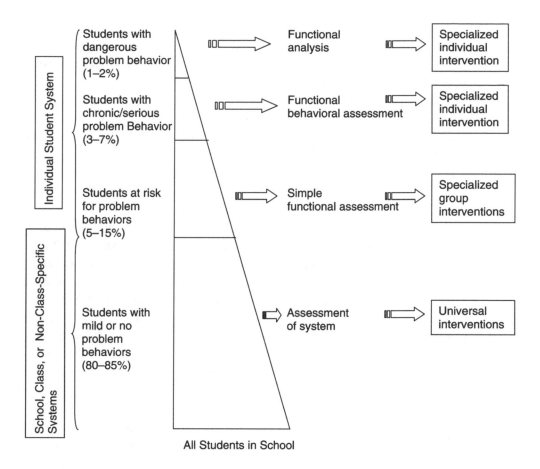

FIGURE 2.4. Continuum of effective behavioral assessment and support. Copyright 2003 by Deanne A. Crone and Robert H. Horner. Based on Walker, et al. (1996).

get a new behavior card and demonstrate that he or she has all the necessary materials for the day. Throughout the day, the student's teachers rate the extent to which the student has met his or her behavioral goals (ratings are usually on a scale of 0–2). At the end of the day, each student "checks out" with the educational assistant and leaves a copy of the daily behavior card. This same system is applied to all the identified at-risk students. If the data (from daily behavior card ratings) indicate that the system is ineffective for a particular child, a simple FBA can be conducted to determine strategies for individualizing the targeted-group intervention for the child. The most important consideration will be whether or not the targeted-group intervention matches the function of the student's problem behavior. We expect that a targeted-group intervention or a simple FBA will be adequate for slightly more than half of the referrals to the individual-student system.

Approximately one-third of the "top of the triangle students" (or 3–7% of the total school population) will be individual students with serious problem behaviors. Many of these students may be at risk for suspension or expulsion. These students will require a full FBA and an individualized BSP.

Typically, less than 15% of the individual student system referrals (or 1–2 % of the school population) will involve students with severe, chronic, or dangerous behaviors. These students may be at risk for expulsion, at risk for alternative school placement, or may be a danger to themselves or others. The Behavior Support Team will need to devote more resources and time to assessment and intervention for these students. A functional analysis of behavior may be appropriate for this small segment of the team's referrals.

The amount of time, resources, and analysis invested in FBA will depend on the comprehensiveness of the assessment. We estimate that a simple FBA will last roughly 20–30 minutes. A full FBA (as defined in this book) will require approximately 2 hours, and a functional analysis can consume as much as 20 or more hours of staff time (Gable, 1999; Gresham, Quinn, & Restori, 1999). Additional time will be required to design, implement, and monitor the BSP. The actual amount of time invested will vary from school to school. Regardless of interschool differences, the time commitment is increased considerably as one moves from a simple FBA to a full FBA to a functional analysis.

• *Does the three-tiered model of responding to individual behavior referrals meet IDEA standards?* The answer is yes. The amendments to IDEA (1997) require that "in response to certain disciplinary actions by school personnel, the IEP team must, within 10 days, meet to formulate a functional behavioral assessment plan to collect data for developing a behavior intervention plan, or if a behavior intervention plan already exists, the team must review and revise it (as necessary), to ensure that it addresses the behavior upon which disciplinary action is predicated." *In other words, schools are required to conduct a full FBA for any student with a disability who is at risk for suspension (greater than 10 days in one school year), expulsion, or alternative school placement.* Many of the students referred to the Behavior Support Team will not meet these criteria. For such students, a simple FBA may suffice. In a court of law, a simple FBA is unlikely to meet the requirements of IDEA (1997) for students who *do* meet the criteria listed above. Both the full FBA and the functional analysis meet these requirements.

Utilizing a function-based approach (i.e., simple FBA, full FBA, functional analysis) at each level of problem severity ensures adherence to standards of professional practice and increases the school's ability to reduce problem behavior and promote appropriate behavior. Figure 2.5 illustrates the decision-making process for deciding between simple FBA, full FBA, and functional analysis.

Decision rule:	Decision rule:	Decision rule:
The student poses a danger to him- or herself or others OR prior assessments were unclear or ineffective.	The student is at risk for a change in placement OR the team has minimal confidence in its hypothesis statement.	The student does not pose a danger, is not at risk for change of placement, AND the team is confident in the hypothesis statement.
Decision:	Decision:	Decision:
Conduct functional analysis	Conduct full functional behavioral assessment	Conduct simple functional behavioral assessment

Meets IDEA (1997) Requirements

Meets Standards of Good Professional Practic

FIGURE 2.5. Decision rules for level of Functional Behavioral Assessment.

• *What steps are involved in conducting a functional behavioral assessment?* An FBA is initiated after the Behavior Support Team receives a request for assistance. The request for assistance can be made by a teacher, an administrator, a team member, a family member, a student, or any other key individuals. The goals, tools, and time investment involved at each level of FBA are outlined in Table 2.1

Simple Functional Behavioral Assessment

The first task is to define the challenge. The Behavior Support Team must build an operational definition of the problem behavior. They will also identify the predictors and consequences of the problem behavior. Often, these tasks can be accomplished in a brief interview with the teacher. Teachers can be the team's greatest resource. Teachers work with and observe their students every day. With focused prompting and practice, the teacher can provide a wealth of information about the predictors, consequences, and underlying functions of problem behavior.

The next step is to use the interview data to generate a testable hypothesis about why the behavior is occurring. The testable hypothesis describes the problem behavior, the predictors and consequences of the problem behavior, and the hypothesized function of the problem behavior. For example, *"When James is asked to read a difficult passage out loud, he throws his books on the floor and swears at the teacher in order to be sent to the office and escape the embarrassment of making a reading error in front of his friends."*

TABLE 2.1. Goals, Process, Tools and Time Investment for Each Level of Functional Assessment

Level of assessment	Goal	Process	Tools	Investment
Simple Functional Behavioral Assessment	Define challenge	Short interview	F-BSP Protocol: Teacher Interview[a] only	20–30 min
			or	
			FACTS-A[b] FACTS-B[c]	20 min
Full Functional Behavioral Assessment	Build understanding of when, how, and why problem behavior occurs	Short interviews	F-BSP Protocol: Teacher/ Parent/Student Interview[a]	20–30 min
			SDFA[d]	20–30 min
		Extended interviews	FA Interview[e]	20–45 min
		Direct observations	FAO[f] FBA form[g]	30 min – 4 hrs
		Review archival records	School records	30 min
Functional Analysis	Confirm understanding	Direct observations and Systematic experimental manipulations	FAO	Up to 20 or more hours

Note. The forms listed should be taken as suggestions. Different forms are available and used by different school districts. Copies of each of the forms listed in Table 2.1 are provided in the Appendices.
[a]Function-Based Behavior Support Plan Protocol; [b]Functional Assessment Checklist for Teachers and Staff—Part A; [c]Functional Assessment Checklist for Teachers and Staff—Part B; [d]Student-Directed Functional Assessment; [e]Functional Assessment Interview (O'Neill et al., 1997); [f]Functional Assessment Observation Form; [g]Functional Behavioral Assessment Observation Form.

Once the initial hypothesis statement is generated, the team decides if they have adequately assessed the problem behavior or if they require additional information: *How confident are they that the hypothesis statement is an accurate explanation for the problem behavior? How serious would the consequences be if they were wrong?* If the team has minimal confidence in their hypothesis statement, they should collect additional assessment information—that is, they should conduct a full FBA. Additionally, if the referred student is at risk of suspension, expulsion, or alternative school placement, the team should invest additional time and resources in the assessment process.

If the team is confident about its hypothesis statement, and the problem behavior is neither dangerous nor placing the student's access to education at risk, the team should develop a BSP based on the simple FBA. The referring person takes the recommended solutions of the team and implements the strategies with the support of team members. A follow-up date is scheduled to evaluate the effectiveness of the recommended strategies.

Full Functional Behavioral Assessment

This is the process of building and testing hypotheses about the problem behavior. The purpose of the full FBA is to improve the effectiveness and efficiency of BSPs. Direct observations and extended interviews are added to the simple FBA. Observations are conducted in the settings where problem behavior typically occurs. At least one observation should be peer-referenced—that is, the identified student's behavior is compared to the behavior of a composite of his peers. Without a peer-referenced comparison, it is difficult to determine if the frequency and intensity of the student's problem behavior is significantly discrepant from his peers. Observations should also document predictors and consequences for each problem behavior event.

The full FBA may also include additional interview data. The student, the parents, and other staff members may be interviewed to provide a more detailed understanding of the problem. (Samples of observation and interview tools are included in the Appendices.) A full FBA may also include a review of academic records.

After completing the full FBA, the team confirms or modifies the testable hypothesis. If the team feels unsure that they have accurately identified the predictors, consequences, and function of the problem behavior with the FBA, they must make another decision. *Should they design a BSP based on the FBA, or should they invest a significant amount of time and resources to conduct a functional analysis?*

This decision must be made without capriciousness. A functional analysis is likely to consume significantly more hours and will require the assistance of personnel with expertise in applied behavior analysis. The team must decide if they have the resources available for conducting a functional analysis in each case. If resources are readily available, the Behavior Support Team can go ahead with the functional analysis. If resources are sparse, the Behavior Support Team must first consider the severity of the consequences of being wrong about their testable hypothesis, and choose to conduct or not conduct a functional analysis, accordingly. For example, if the student poses a significant danger to himself or others, a functional analysis of his behavior may be warranted. If a functional analysis is not recommended, the team will begin to design the BSP. (In many cases, it will be reasonable to decide to design and test a BSP at this point.)

Functional Analysis

The functional analysis allows the team to empirically confirm their understanding of the problem behavior, predictors, and functions. Functional analysis involves the experimental, systematic manipulation of environmental variables to evaluate hypothesis statements (Vollmer & Northrup, 1996). The functional analysis should result in a clear understanding of the predictors, maintaining consequences, and function of the problem behavior. This information is used in the design and implementation of the BSP.

The reader may note that the assessment period is the longest for the cases with the most severe consequences. The assessment period is increased from 20–30 minutes to 2 hours, and then from 2 hours to as many as 20 hours or more. In cases of serious behavioral consequences, the teacher will not have the luxury to wait through several hours' worth of assessment. Teachers need an intermediary plan for addressing immediate problem behavior. Schools should have a universal crisis plan for dealing with serious problem behaviors. While the Behavior Support Team completes the FBA, the school should support the teacher with a short-term crisis plan for keeping the student and the classroom safe (refer to the Supplementary Section in Chapter 1 for resources on crisis plans).

INTERVENTION

- *What steps are involved in evaluating and modifying a behavior support plan?* Once the team has decided on and completed the appropriate level of FBA, they begin the process of designing, implementing, and modifying the BSP. The BSP should produce multiple outcomes: (1) procedures for preventing the problem behavior through alteration of the setting events and predictors; (2) procedures for teaching appropriate behaviors; (3) procedures for manipulating consequences of problem behaviors; (4) consideration of the contextual fit of the BSP; (5) data-collection procedures for evaluating the effectiveness of the BSP; and (6) a timeline for implementation, evaluation, and follow-up.

Table 2.2 lists the procedures involved in designing a BSP. Additionally, examples of hypothetical BSPs are given in Chapter 4. For additional information on designing BSPs, refer to the basic texts listed in the Supplementary Section of Chapter 1.

After the BSP is implemented, the Behavior Support Team must evaluate the plan in terms of its effectiveness and efficiency. The team should reconvene 2–3 weeks after the initiation of the BSP. The team should then review the goals of the BSP, examine the behavioral data, and determine if the goals have been met. If the goals have been achieved, the next step is to evaluate the efficiency of the

TABLE 2.2. Steps and Procedures for Designing a Behavior Support Plan

Problem identification

- Receive request for assistance
- Decide to build formal plan of support

Functional Behavioral Assessment

- Describe problem behaviors in operational terms
- Conduct interview and observations to build and test hypothesis statements
- Conduct functional analysis if necessary

Design Plan of Support

- Generate behavioral goals
- Complete the Build a Competing Behavior Pathway form (see Appendix B, Step 6)
- Generate a list of potential intervention strategies
- Consider all relevant contextual variables
- Select elements of BSP

Implement Plan

- Agree on the roles and responsibilities of each individual on team
- Agree on the roles and responsibilities of additional key players (e.g., parents, student)
- Decide on a time for follow-up meeting
- Document the intervention plan in a BSP
- Distribute BSP to all participating individuals
- Implement BSP

BSP. *Is the BSP adequately efficient or can it be redesigned to save time and re-sources?* If the efficiency of the BSP is adequate, the team does not need to modify or reevaluate it. They should plan to conduct a follow-up meeting for the student in 2–6 months. If the efficiency of the BSP can be improved, the team decides on the necessary modifications. The modified BSP is implemented. After 2–3 weeks, the team should meet again to reevaluate the effectiveness and efficiency of the modified BSP.

In the original evaluation meeting (2–3 weeks after initiation of the original plan), the team may decide that the goals have not been achieved. Prior to making modifications to the BSP, the team needs to determine the reason why the goals were not achieved. Very commonly, the BSP is ineffective because it is not implemented appropriately. The team should consider if there are contextual limitations that make it difficult to implement the plan (contextual limitations will be discussed further in Chapter 4). If there are serious contextual limitations, the team should take these into consideration and modify the plan. If there are no contextual limitations, the BSP should be reimplemented with fidelity.

The team may find that the goals of the BSP were not achieved despite adequate implementation of the plan. The BSP may have been unsuccessful because the original assessment of the problem behavior was incorrect. The team must decide if further FBA is necessary. Further assessment may be appropriate, especially if the original BSP was based on data from a simple FBA. If the Behavior Support Team decides that further assessment is needed, they should continue to build and confirm an understanding of the problem through additional observations, interviews, or systematic manipulations. If the team feels that further FBA is not necessary, they should make modifications to the BSP. Once again, they should plan to reconvene in 2–3 weeks to evaluate the effectiveness and efficiency of the plan. The steps involved in a simple FBA, a full FBA, and functional analysis are summarized in the flow chart in Figure 2.6.

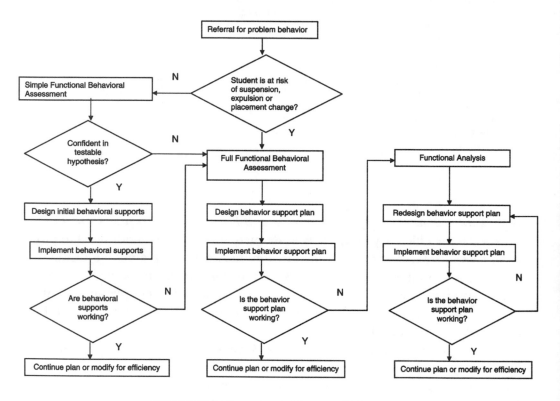

FIGURE 2.6. Flow chart of the FBA-BSP process.

PART TWO

Embedding Functional Behavioral Assessment within School Systems: Case Examples

CHAPTER 3

Conducting a Functional
Behavioral Assessment

INTRODUCTION

This chapter begins a detailed illustration of the FBA-BSP process as it would occur in a school. The emphasis in the chapter is on simple FBA and full FBA, not
functional analysis. For references on functional analysis, turn to the Supplementary Section of this chapter. To illustrate the FBA-BSP process, case vignettes
of three students were chosen and serve as a cross section of exemplars. The following vignettes do not represent real children, but rather were created as examples to demonstrate the FBA-BSP process across a range of students.

Case Example 1

Tom is a third-grade student in a general education classroom. Tom transferred to his current school in the middle of the academic year. Tom was referred to the Behavior Support Team by his teacher for fighting, verbal ha-
rassment of other students, and being disrespectful to adults. Tom has a
very short temper. He has some academic difficulties in reading and writing,
and he works with a reading resource teacher for 1.5 hours per week. Tom
is athletic and enjoys leading sport activities during recess.

Case Example 2

Vera is a kindergarten student who loves to be the center of adult attention.
She has a quick temper. She frequently talks out in class. She also frequently
"tattles" on other students. When other students use materials that are
meant to be shared, she yells at them, tells the teacher, and starts to cry and

scream. During recess she has pushed other children on the ground when they have made her angry. Vera's parents recently divorced. In the first 6 months of kindergarten, Vera has been referred to the office 10 times for her temper tantrums and other problem behavior.

Case Example 3

Ronald is a 12-year-old boy in seventh grade who is disruptive and physically aggressive. He has a diagnosis of Attention-Deficit/Hyperactivity Disorder and is taking Ritalin twice a day. As a third grader, Ronald was referred for special education services due to his poor academic performance and frequent behavior problems. In the first 20 weeks of school, Ronald received over 50 discipline referrals. At the time of referral to the individual Behavior Support Team, the school was considering expelling him from school for his problem behavior.

THE ASSESSMENT PROCESS

The assessment process begins with a referral to the Behavior Support Team. Typically, a teacher makes the referral, but the referral can also begin with a parent or a nonteaching staff member, such as the lunchroom monitor. The referral is given to the referral liaison/coordinator. The liaison/coordinator routes the referral to the Behavior Support Team, who begin the FBA-BSP process. A sample of a completed referral form for each of the case examples is presented in Figures 3.1, 3.2, and 3.3. A blank Request for Assistance Form is included in Appendix A. (In the sample, only page one of the form is used. A question regarding expected behavior has been added to page one.)

As the coordinator examines the teacher referral for each of these students, she or he may note important details that will be informative to the FBA-BSP process. For example, the teachers for both Vera (Figure 3.1) and Ronald (Figure 3.3) have relied heavily on "punishment procedures," such as detention, office referrals, reprimands, and discipline-related communication with parents. Although each teacher has been trying these punishment strategies *"since school started,"* they have *"not yet seen any change in behavior." "Discipline doesn't seem to faze this child."*

These Requests for Assistance Forms illustrate five important points. First, these reactive responses are not working. The BSP will have to incorporate a different, more proactive approach to managing the problem behavior. Second, the level of stress or exasperation experienced by the teacher is often evident on the Request for Assistance Form. The comments of Ronald's teacher in response to the question regarding strategy use demonstrate a high degree of frustration. This is a teacher who will need a great deal of support in the initial stages of im-

Request for Assistance Form

Date 1/4/99 _____   Teacher/Team Ms. Rlley _____
                                 IEP: Yes No (Circle)
Student Name Vera _____ Grade K-garten _____

Situations	Problem Behaviors	Most Common Result
Aggression is unpredictable	Talk-outs Pushing She's a tattle-tale	Other students get upset I talk with her about how her behavior is not the way that kindergartners behave

What have you tried/used? How has it worked?
All the time I tell her not to tattle. She has been sent to office for pushing and the referrals last a half-hour, and I talked to her mom. I've been doing this since school started but have not yet seen any change in behavior. I'll keep trying, but it's not working!

What is your behavioral goal/expectation for this student? Don't tattle _____

What have you tried to date to change the situations in which the problem behavior(s) occur?

___ Modified assignments to match the student's skills	X Changed seating assignments	___ Changed schedule of activities	Other?
___ Arranged tutoring to improve the student's academic skills	___ Changed curriculum	___ Provided extra assistance	

What have you tried to date to teach expected behaviors?

X Reminders about expected behavior when problem behavior is likely	___ Clarified rules and expected behavior for the whole class	___ Practiced the expected behaviors in class	Other?
___ Reward program for expected behavior	X Oral agreement with the student	___ Self-management program	
___ Systematic feedback about behavior	___ Individual written contract with the student	___ Contract with student/ with parents	

What consequences have you tried to date for the problem behavior?

X Loss of privileges	X Note or phone call to the student's parents	X Office referral	Other?
___ Time-out	___ Detention	X Reprimand	
___ Referral to school counselor	___ Meeting with the student's parents	___ Individual meeting with the student	

FIGURE 3.1. Request for assistance—Vera. The form itself is adapted from Todd, Horner, Sugai, and Colvin (1999). Copyright 1999 by Lawrence Erlbaum Associates. Adapted by permission.

Request for Assistance Form

Date _10/5/98_   Teacher/Team _Ms. Smith_
                                                 IEP: Yes No (Circle)

Student Name _Tom_   Grade _3rd_

Situations	Problem Behaviors	Most Common Result
Mostly in class Not on playground or cafeteria Whenever I ask him to do something he doesn't want to do	Fighting Calls other students names Pushes adults Talks back to adults	Gets into arguments with adults or other students Gets an office referral

What have you tried/used? How has it worked?
I give him office referrals and reprimands. In October, I put him in a reading group that is at his level and gave him one-to-one help in reading. The changes in reading group seem to be the most effective. I'll keep working on his reading skills and will keep giving office referrals until they work.

What is your behavioral goal/expectation for this student? _Don't be disrespectful to others_

What have you tried to date to change the situations in which the problem behavior(s) occur?

X Modified assignments to match the student's skills	X Changed seating assignments	___ Changed schedule of activities	Other?
___ Arranged tutoring to improve the student's academic skills	X Changed curriculum	X Provided extra assistance	

What have you tried to date to teach expected behaviors?

X Reminders about expected behavior when problem behavior is likely	___ Clarified rules and expected behavior for the whole class	___ Practiced the expected behaviors in class	Other?
___ Reward program for expected behavior	X Oral agreement with the student	___ Self-management program	
___ Systematic feedback about behavior	___ Individual written contract with the student	___ Contract with student/ with parents	

What consequences have you tried to date for the problem behavior?

___ Loss of privileges	___ Note or phone call to the student's parents	X Office referral	Other?
___ Time-out	___ Detention	X Reprimand	
___ Referral to school counselor	___ Meeting with the student's parents	___ Individual meeting with the student	

FIGURE 3.2. Request for assistance—Tom. The form itself is adapted from Todd, Horner, Sugai, and Colvin (1999). Copyright 1999 by Lawrence Erlbaum Associates. Adapted by permission.

Request for Assistance Form

Date 2/1/99

Teacher/Team Mr. Jackson

IEP: Yes No (Circle)

Student Name Ronald

Grade 7th

Situations	Problem Behaviors	Most Common Result
Happens all the time Just seems to come out of the blue	Aggressive and out-of-control bullying	I tell him over and over to behave himself. The kids end up ignoring him. He gets referrals and suspension

What have you tried/used? How has it worked?
Since the beginning of the year I have tried detention, discipline referrals, notes to parents, reprimands, and suspensions. Discipline doesn't seem to faze this child and I'm tired of telling this student to behave!

What is your behavioral goal/expectation for this student? Don't fight

What have you tried to date to change the situations in which the problem behavior(s) occur?

___ Modified assignments to match the student's skills	X Changed seating assignments	___ Changed schedule of activities	Other?
___ Arranged tutoring to improve the student's academic skills	___ Changed curriculum	___ Provided extra assistance	

What have you tried to date to teach expected behaviors?

X Reminders about expected behavior when problem behavior is likely	X Clarified rules and expected behavior for the whole class	___ Practiced the expected behaviors in class	Other?
___ Reward program for expected behavior	___ Oral agreement with the student	___ Self-management program	
___ Systematic feedback about behavior	___ Individual written contract with the student	___ Contract with student/ with parents	

What consequences have you tried to date for the problem behavior?

X Loss of privileges	X Note or phone call to the student's parents	X Office referral	Other?
___ Time-out	X Detention	X Reprimand	
X Referral to school counselor	___ Meeting with the student's parents	___ Individual meeting with the student	

FIGURE 3.3. Request for assistance—Ronald. The form itself is adapted from Todd, Horner, Sugai, and Colvin (1999). Copyright 1999 by Lawrence Erlbaum Associates. Adapted by permission.

plementation of the BSP. Third, it is important to note that the teachers believe that if they keep persisting on these ineffective strategies, eventually the strategies will work: *"I'll keep trying, but it's not working"*; *"I'll . . . keep giving office referrals until they work."*

Despite evidence to the contrary, teachers often exhibit a great deal of faith in punishment as the most effective strategy for behavior change. Even in the face of continued failure, they often continue to use punishment strategies as the strategy of choice. The coordinator and the Behavior Support Team will need to work with the referring teachers to help them explore and understand alternative strategies for behavior change.

Tom's teacher has relied somewhat on punishment strategies, but has also tried curriculum modifications to attempt to reduce the student's problem behaviors (Figure 3.2). The teacher has seen some success in these efforts. The Behavior Support Team should determine the extent to which they can build on some of these effective strategies. They should also encourage and support the teacher for successful efforts thus far.

Further analysis of the Request for Assistance Forms illustrates a fourth important point: the teachers' description of problem behavior is rather vague and uninformative. Vera is described as a *"tattle-tale,"* Ronald as *"aggressive"* and *"out-of-control."* These descriptors do not provide an observable, measurable description of the problem behavior. The teachers have been unable to identify the times that the behavior is most likely to occur. To the teachers, the behavior seems to occur *"all the time,"* or it is *"unpredictable"* and *"out of the blue."* The team will have to work with teachers to develop an *operational definition* of the problem and to determine the most common predictors of the problem behavior.

An operational definition of problem behavior describes behavior in observable, measurable terms. The description of the behavior should be so explicit that two observers could independently observe a student and agree on whether or not the behavior had occurred. For example, rather than describing Ronald as "aggressive," the teacher could say, "Ronald hits other students in the arm with enough force to hurt the other student" or "Ronald kicks the legs of his chair and the chairs of other students around him."

The concepts of operationally defining behaviors and identifying predictors will be foreign at first to many teachers. After enough opportunities to use behavioral assessment terminology, teachers will become more fluent in defining problem behaviors and identifying predictors and consequences. The Behavior Support Team will begin to see a significant difference in the quality of information communicated in the Request for Assistance Form. Compare the Request for Assistance Form for Ronald to the one for Tom. Tom's teacher has been at the school for 8 years. In the course of the past 3 years, she has requested assistance for four students. In contrast, Ronald's teacher is a first-year teacher. This is the first time he has needed to manage the problem behavior of a difficult student. There is a distinct difference in the clarity of the information reported.

Finally, the coordinator may notice that many of the expected behaviors are listed as negative rules—*"don't fight"* and *"don't tattle."* Adults must *teach students to perform expected behaviors* in addition to informing them about which behaviors are not allowed. Explicitly teaching expectations to students provides them with an alternative behavior to replace the inappropriate behavior. For example, *"keep hands and feet to self"* and *"be respectful"* are two rules that inform students of expected behaviors. In developing the BSP, the team can help the teacher identify how to define, teach, and reward expected behaviors.

Simple Functional Behavioral Assessment (Simple FBA)

The next step in the process is to conduct the simple FBA. The simple FBA consists of a brief interview with the student's primary teacher. (Middle school and high school students typically do not have a primary teacher. In this case, the interview should be conducted with the referring teacher.) The simple FBA acknowledges and relies on the wealth of information that an individual teacher has about his or her student. The major purposes of the interview are to (1) identify the problem behaviors, (2) define important characteristics of the problem behaviors, (3) identify times of day when problem behaviors are most likely to occur, (4) identify common predictors and setting events for problem behaviors, and (5) identify typical consequences of problem behaviors that impact reoccurrence of problem behavior.

Teacher Interview

The Behavior Support Team can choose to use any teacher interview with which they are familiar, if it provides the necessary FBA information. The Functional Behavioral Assessment-Behavior Support Plan Protocol (F-BSP Protocol) draws heavily from the Functional Assessment Checklist for Teachers (FACTS; March et al., 2000), and was developed to include, among other things, a teacher interview instrument that meets the previously listed objectives. This interview instrument is efficient, easy to use, and easy to train to use. Figures 3.4, 3.5, and 3.6 illustrate completed teacher interview forms for each of the three case examples. Please note that the teacher interview is one part of the entire F-BSP Protocol. Each part of the protocol is demonstrated throughout Chapters 3, 4, and 5. A complete, blank, F-BSP Protocol, along with instructions for its use, is included in Appendix B.

Typically, the teacher interview is administered by a member of the Behav-

FUNCTIONAL BEHAVIORAL ASSESSMENT INTERVIEW—
TEACHER/STAFF/PARENT

Student Name Vera   **Age:** 5   **Grade:** K   **Date:** 1/6/99
Person(s) interviewed: Ms. Riley (teacher)
Interviewer: Mr. Kohn (Action Team member)

Student Profile: What is the student good at or what are some strengths that the student brings to school?
Very sensitive and caring towards adults and her baby brother, speaks up for herself

---

Step 1A: Interview Teacher/Staff/Parent

Description of the Behavior

> **What does the problem behavior(s) look like?**
> If another child wants to share her materials, she will get mad, tell on the student, cry, and be aggressive enough to get the materials back
>
> **How often does the problem behavior(s) occur?**
> 3–4 times a week
>
> **How long does the problem behavior(s) last when it does occur?**
> 1–5 minutes
>
> **How disruptive or dangerous is the problem behavior(s)?**
> Not too dangerous, but is disruptive to the teacher

Description of the Antecedent
Identifying Routines: When, where, and with whom are problem behaviors most likely?

Schedule (Times)	Activity	Specific Problem Behavior	Likelihood of Problem Behavior	With Whom Does Problem Occur?
9:00	Attendance, personal activity		Low High 1 ②3 4 5 6	
9:15	Circle time in large group	Tattles, pushes, whines	1 2 3 4 ⑤6	Peers
9:45	Snack	Tattles, pushes, whines	1 2 ③4 5 6	
10:00	Sounds/leters in large group	Tattles, pushes, whines	1 2 3 ④5 6	Peers
10:20	Art/music in large group	Tattles, pushes, whines	1 2 3 4 ⑤6	Peers
10:50	Recess	Tattles, pushes, whines	1 2 3 ④5 6	Peers
11:05	Small-group activities	Tattles, pushes, whines	1 2 ③4 5 6	Peers
11:30	Dismissal		1 ②3 4 5 6	

(continued)

FIGURE 3.4. Completed teacher interview—Vera. The form itself is adapted by permission from March et al. (2000).

Summarize Antecedent (and Setting Events)

> **What situations seem to set off the problem behavior?** (difficult tasks, transitions, structured activities, small-group settings, teacher's request, particular individuals, etc.)
> Happens both during structured time and unstructured activities—any time that there is more than one student working near or with her. Task difficulty does not seem to influence the behavior.
>
> **When is the problem behavior most likely to occur?** (times of day and days of the week)
> Circle time (Large group); art or music (Large group); or recess
>
> **When is the problem behavior least likely to occur?** (times of day and days of the week)
> Attendance in the morning/personal activity time, dismissal
>
> **Setting Events: Are there specific conditions, events, or activities that make the problem behavior worse?** (missed medication, history of academic failure, conflict at home, missed meals, lack of sleep, history of problems with peers, etc.)
> If she has a bad morning on the bus and comes in to school upset.

Description of the Consequence

> **What usually happens after the behavior occurs?** (what is the teacher's reaction, how do other students react, is the student sent to the office, does the student get out of doing work, does the student get in a power struggle, etc.)
> Other kids usually back off and allow her to get the materials she wants. Teacher talks with her about how it is not nice to tattle. Teacher often talks with mother and mother talks to her about the tattling. On occasion she has been sent to the office because she has had a tantrum in the class—crying, yelling at other kids, ripping up the picture another student was working on.

- - - - - - End of Interview - - - - - -

Step 2A: Propose a Testable Explanation

Setting Event	Antecedent	Behavior	Consequence
Difficult morning at home or on bus	Large-group setting with peers, when expected to share materials	1. Tattles, pushes, whines, and cries	Teacher talks to her about appropriate behavior. Mother talks to her at home. Obtains desired materials from peers.

Function of the Behavior

For each ABC sequence listed above, why do you think the behavior is occurring? (to get teacher attention, to get peer attention, gets desired object/activity, escapes undesirable activity, escapes demand, escapes particular people, etc.)

1. Vera seems to be having the tantrums to get adult attention and to get access to the materials she wants._

How confident are you that your testable explanation is accurate?

Very sure			So-so		Not at all sure
6	5	4	③	2	1

FIGURE 3.4. *(continued)*

FUNCTIONAL BEHAVIORAL ASSESSMENT INTERVIEW—
TEACHER/STAFF/PARENT

Student Name: Tom   **Age:** 8   **Grade:** 3   **Date:** 10/7/99
Person(s) interviewed: Ms. Smith (teacher
Interviewer: Miss Sand (Action Team member)

Student Profile: What is the student good at or what are some strengths that the student brings to school?
Very athletic, a leader on the playground, other students seek him out to be on their team

Step 1A: Interview Teacher/Staff/Parent

Description of the Behavior

What does the problem behavior(s) look like?
He gets frustrated, refuses to work, throws his books down, tries to push the "teacher's buttons" by yelling and teasing.
How often does the problem behavior(s) occur?
Big tantrums occur 2–3 times a week, at some point in the morning.
Smaller displays of frustration and work refusal occur almost daily.
How long does the problem behavior(s) last when it does occur?
Big tantrums—seems to build for about an hour or more until lunch time.
Other times he has brief tantrums, but they reoccur more frequently, whenever he is redirected.
How disruptive or dangerous is the problem behavior(s)?
Detrimental to his academic progress. Disturbs whole class, has caused bruises from pushing.

Description of the Antecedent
Identifying Routines: When, where, and with whom are problem behaviors most likely?

Schedule (Times)	Activity	Specific Problem Behavior	Likelihood of Problem Behavior	With Whom Does Problem Occur?
			Low High	
8:45	Attendance and sharing		1 ② 3 4 5 6	
9:00	Math	Refuses to work Shouts at teacher	1 2 3 4 ⑤ 6	Teacher aide
9:45	Music/art/social studies	Slams things on desk	1 2 3 4 ⑤ 6	Teacher
10:15	Unstructured study period	Pushes peers	1 2 3 ④ 5 6	Peers and teacher
10:45	Recess		① 2 3 4 5 6	
11:00	Reading		1 2 ③ 4 5 6	Peers and teacher
12:00	Lunch		① 2 3 4 5 6	
12:45	Spelling		1 2 ③ 4 5 6	Teacher
1:00	Language arts		1 2 3 ④ 5 6	Teacher
2:00	Recess		① 2 3 4 5 6	
2:15	Science		1 2 ③ 4 5 6	Peers and teacher

(continued)

FIGURE 3.5. Completed teacher interview—Tom. The form itself is adapted by permission from March et al. (2000).

Summarize Antecedent (and Setting Events)

> **What situations seem to set off the problem behavior?** (difficult tasks, transitions, structured activities, small-group settings, teacher's request, particular individuals, etc.)
> Big tantrums—structured time, academically difficult, before recess, negative peer interactions
> Brief frustration/noncompliance—difficult task with no 1:1 aide
>
> **When is the problem behavior most likely to occur?** (times of day and days of the week)
> Big tantrums—Math or 9:45–10:15 period
> Brief frustration—Language Arts, Study period, Reading, Spelling, Science
>
> **When is the problem behavior least likely to occur?** (times of day and days of the week)
> Recess, Lunch, Attendance, & Sharing
>
> **Setting Events: Are there specific conditions, events, or activities that make the problem behavior worse?** (missed medication, history of academic failure, conflict at home, missed meals, lack of sleep, history of problems with peers, etc.)
> He has a history of academic failure. Behavior is worse if the 1:1 aide cannot come in that day

Description of the Consequence

> **What usually happens after the behavior occurs?** (what is the teacher's reaction, how do other students react, is the student sent to the office, does the student get out of doing work, does the student get in a power struggle, etc.)
> Behavior is disturbing enough that the class stops. Other kids tell him to be quiet and the teacher also reprimands him. Sometimes he is sent to the office. Often times he ends up not doing any work the whole class period.

- - - - - - End of Interview - - - - - -

Step 2A: Propose a Testable Explanation

Setting Event	Antecedent	Behavior	Consequence
1:1 aide absent	During structured time that occurs before recess, Peer makes comment to him	1. Refuses to work, shouts, slams books, disturbs other students	Teacher attention, peer attention
History of academic failure	Difficult academic tasks to do without an aide	2. Refuse to work, slams books	Teacher attention, gets out of doing work

Function of the Behavior

For each ABC sequence listed above, why do you think the behavior is occurring? (to get teacher attention, to get peer attention, gets desired object/activity, escapes undesirable activity, escapes demand, escapes particular people, etc.)

1. Tom is having the big tantrums in order to get peer attention and teacher attention
2. Tom is having smaller tantrums/work refusal in order to escape tasks that he htinks he can't do on his own and to get teacher attention

How confident are you that your testable explanation is accurate?

Very sure			So-so		Not at all sure
6	5	4	③	2	1

FIGURE 3.5. (continued)

FUNCTIONAL BEHAVIORAL ASSESSMENT INTERVIEW—
TEACHER/STAFF/PARENT

Student Name Ronald _____ **Age:** 13 **Grade:** 7 **Date:** 2/3/99
Person(s) interviewed: Mr. Jackson (teacher) _____
Interviewer: Mrs. Andrews (Action Team member) _____

Student Profile: What is the student good at or what are some strengths that the student brings to school?
Comes to school every day _____

Step 1A: Interview Teacher/Staff/Parent

Description of the Behavior

What does the problem behavior(s) look like?
Can't work well in groups. If someone makes a remark to him, he gets mad and punches the student, usually in the arm. He holds grudges and will often fight after school.
Also yells at teacher and refuses to do work.

How often does the problem behavior(s) occur?
Fighting, about once a week.
Work refusal, every class period. Yelling at teacher, approximately twice a week.

How long does the problem behavior(s) last when it does occur?
Fighting in class lasts about 5–10 minutes.
Work refusal lasts most of class period unless sent to office. Yelling is brief but reoccurring.

How disruptive or dangerous is the problem behavior(s)?
Fighting is dangerous. He has sent another student to the nurse with a bloody nose.
Yelling is disruptive to class and teacher. Work refusal has put him in danger of failing seventh grade.

Description of the Antecedent
Identifying Routines: When, where, and with whom are problem behaviors most likely?

Schedule (Times)	Activity	Specific Problem Behavior	Likelihood of Problem Behavior	With Whom Does Problem Occur?
			Low High	
8:20–9:15	Science	Fighting	1 2 3 ④ 5 6	Peers
9:20–10:15	Math	Yelling, work refusal	1 2 3 4 5 ⑥	Teacher
10:20–11:15	Reading	Yelling, work refusal	1 2 3 4 5 ⑥	Teacher
11:20–12:15	Spanish	Yelling, work refusal	1 2 3 4 ⑤ 6	Teacher
12:20–1:00	Lunch		① 2 3 4 5 6	
1:05–2:00	Social Studies	Fighting	1 2 3 ④ 5 6	Peers
2:05–3:00	Physical Education		① 2 3 4 5 6	

(continued)

FIGURE 3.6. Completed teacher interview—Ronald. The form itself is adapted by permission from March et al. (2000).

Summarize Antecedent (and Setting Events)

What situations seem to set off the problem behavior? (difficult tasks, transitions, structured activities, small-group settings, teacher's request, particular individuals, etc.)
Fighting—most frequent when he is doing group work, especially with certain students.
Work refusal/yelling—when asked to complete assignments in class, that are long or difficult.

When is the problem behavior most likely to occur? (times of day and days of the week)
Fighting—Science and Social Studies
Work refusal/yelling—Math, Reading, and Spanish

When is the problem behavior least likely to occur? (times of day and days of the week)
No problems during lunch or physical education.

Setting Events: Are there specific conditions, events, or activities that make the problem behavior worse? (missed medication, history of academic failure, conflict at home, missed meals, lack of sleep, history of problems with peers, etc.)
Behavior is worse when he is around specific students or when he has been in a fight in the past day or two.

Description of the Consequence

What usually happens after the behavior occurs? (what is the teacher's reaction, how do other students react, is the student sent to the office, does the student get out of doing work, does the student get in a power struggle, etc.)
Fighting—other kids back off and tell the teacher, teacher sends him to office.
Work refusal/yelling—often gets away with not doing work, although he engages each teacher in a long verbal battle over it. He is receiving failing grades in many classes.

- - - - - - End of Interview - - - - - -

Step 2A: Propose a Testable Explanation

Setting Event	Antecedent	Behavior	Consequence
Specific classmates, activity not monitored	Expectation to do cooperative group work. Peer makes a negative or neutral comment to him.	1. Becomes angry. Tells classmate to leave him alone. If behavior is allowed to escalate, he'll punch classmate in the arm.	Other students back off. Often gets sent to office.
History of academic failure	Expectation to complete assignment that is difficult/long.	2. Work refusal. Yelling at teacher about the work.	Ends up not working in class. Teacher argues with him. Gets sent to office.

Function of the Behavior

For each ABC sequence listed above, why do you think the behavior is occurring? (to get teacher attention, to get peer attention, gets desired object/activity, escapes undesirable activity, escapes demand, escapes particular people, etc.)

1. Ronald is punching peers to assert authority and thereby escape negative peer interactions

2. Ronald is refusing work and arguing with teacher because it gets him out of doing the work

How confident are you that your testable explanation is accurate?

Very sure			So-so		Not at all sure
6	5	4	③	2	1

FIGURE 3.6. (continued)

ior Support Team. As teachers become more comfortable with the process of FBA, they may complete the interview form without the assistance of a team member. The interview takes approximately 20–30 minutes to complete. This interview form has several advantages as an assessment instrument. First, it eliminates vague descriptions of problem behavior. In order to be useful, descriptions of problem behavior have to be given in such a way that two people looking at the same event will label it as the same problem behavior. For example, there is a meaningful difference between saying *"Lisa is just like a kid with ADHD"* and *"Lisa is disorganized. Her desk is full of crumpled papers. It takes her three times as long as her classmates to find the appropriate book and materials. She rarely sits still for more than 10 minutes. She answers out of turn and interrupts other children and adults."*

The teacher interview from the F-BSP Protocol guides teachers to give useful definitions of problem behaviors by requiring specific, measurable, objective information that describes the frequency, intensity, and context of problem behavior. On the Request for Assistance Form, Vera was described as a *"tattle-tale."* The completed teacher interview (Figure 3.4) provides a much clearer picture of her problematic behavior: i.e., *"If another child wants to share her materials, she will get mad, tell on the student, cry and be aggressive enough to get the materials back."* This happens *"3–4 times a week"* and each episode lasts *"1–5 minutes."* The behavior is *"not too dangerous, but is disruptive to the teacher."*

The second major advantage of the teacher interview from the F-BSP Protocol is that it emphasizes the child's routines, not the child, in identifying the problem. In other words, the interview focuses staff attention on alterable events, the things that the staff members have control over. It guides the team to look for predictors and patterns in the problem behavior and to begin to identify where the most impact can be made. The interview accomplishes this by illustrating those times of day that are problematic for a child and those that are not difficult. For example, on the Request for Assistance Form, Ronald's teacher indicated that his problem behavior *"happens all the time,"* and *"just seems to come out of the blue."* However, the completed F-BSP interview (Figure 3.6) clearly indicates that certain times of the day are much more problematic for Ronald than others. During math and reading there is a very high likelihood that Ronald will engage in problem behavior. Lunch and physical education are relatively problem-free. This information will be critical in forming hypotheses about the problem behavior and in designing effective BSPs.

The final step in completing the teacher interview from the F-BSP Protocol is to develop a testable hypothesis to explain why the problem behavior is occurring. Testable hypotheses are developed for each problematic routine. Many children have complicated patterns of problem behavior, which may require the team to identify several distinct routines.

Developing a Testable Hypothesis

The testable hypothesis serves as a prescription for the BSP, suggesting which predictors and consequences of behavior should be manipulated in order to reduce the problem behavior and indicating which new behaviors should be taught to replace the problem behavior. The testable hypothesis also creates a link between the FBA and the BSP by describing the function served by the problem behavior. Research identifies at least two major function(s) of problem behavior: positive reinforcement and negative reinforcement (Carr, 1977; O'Neill et al., 1997). If problem behaviors are maintained by obtaining something (e.g., attention or a tangible item), the behavior functions as positive reinforcement for the child (O'Neill et al., 1997). In contrast, if problem behaviors are maintained by escaping or avoiding something undesirable, the behavior functions as negative reinforcement for the child (O'Neill et al., 1997). The same topographical behavior may serve different functions for the same child or different functions for different children.

In Tom's case, analysis of the routine matrix (Identifying Routines section of Figure 3.5) and the responses to the Summarize Antecedent questions (Figure 3.5) indicate at least two routines that are highly likely to produce problem behavior: (1) structured class times that are demanding and occur before recess; (2) structured class times that are demanding and do not provide 1:1 assistance. Tom's problem behavior for the first routine can be summarized in the following testable hypothesis: *"During structured time that is academically challenging and occurs before recess, Tom will refuse to work, will shout at the teacher, and will slam his books loudly. This problem behavior is maintained by teacher and peer attention."* The following testable hypotheses were developed for Vera and Ronald, respectively. *"When Vera is in a large-group setting with peers, and a classmate attempts to share her materials, Vera will tattle, push, whine, or cry in an attempt to get attention from the teacher." "During group activities with low supervision and long duration, a negative comment by a peer will incite Ronald to punch the other student. This is done in an attempt to force the student to stop making negative comments."*

At the bottom of the second page of the teacher interview of the F-BSP Protocol, a space is provided to indicate how confident the team is in the testable hypothesis. The rating is made on a scale of 1–6, where 1 equals "Not at all sure" and 6 equals "Very sure." A rating of 4, 5, or 6 indicates that the team feels confident that they understand the routines that predict and maintain the problem behavior. A rating of 1, 2, or 3 indicates that the team is not confident that they understand the problem behavior.

At this point, the simple FBA is complete. If two criteria are met, the team can begin to design the BSP without completing a full FBA: (1) the student is not a student with a disability who is at risk for suspension, expulsion, alternative school placement, or any other disciplinary action that limits the student's access to public education; (2) the team has confidence in the accuracy of the initial testable hypothesis (a confidence rating of 4 or more). If either of these criteria is not met, the team should complete a full FBA.

Full Functional Behavioral Assessment (Full FBA)

Additional Interviews

The full FBA builds directly upon the simple FBA. The full FBA includes observation of the student in a natural setting and additional interviews. The interviews may be conducted with additional teachers, the parents, and/or the identified student. Each of these individuals can add valuable information to the overall understanding of the problem behavior.

The teacher interview of the F-BSP Protocol can be adapted to be used with parents. (An example is given in Figure 3.7.) Keeping the interview focused on school-related concerns can be difficult when interviewing families. Families may be dealing with multiple concerns—for example, poverty, divorce, or drug use—in addition to the child's academic difficulties. The interviewer may be tempted to "try to fix everything" or to gather detailed information on every family historical event that "may be the key to why the child acts this way." It is important to be aware of significant family issues that act as setting events for the problem behavior. To be effective, however, the interviewer must stay focused on those things that are within the school's purview and that are alterable events.

As an example, the family may be going through a divorce that is emotionally difficult for the identified student as well as for the rest of the family. The school does not need to provide divorce counseling, nor should it use the divorce to justify and excuse the child's behavior. However, the school should be aware of the divorce and how it may act as a setting event for distractible, withdrawn, or aggressive behavior. To illustrate, joint custody issues may be relevant. Rules, morning routines, and expectations may vary significantly between each parent's household, thereby creating a difference that could significantly impact the child's school behavior in the morning. An intervention strategy that is within the school's domain and that could reduce the impact of negative setting events is to provide the student with a supportive adult mentor who has consistent daily contact with the child before the school day begins. This adult could check in with the child first thing in the morning, make sure that the child has had something for breakfast, has brought all of his or her school materials, and is ready to begin the day.

An effective strategy for keeping the parent interview focused on school-

FUNCTIONAL BEHAVIORAL ASSESSMENT INTERVIEW—
TEACHER/STAFF/PARENT

Student Name: Tom   **Age:** 8   **Grade:** 3   **Date:** 10/7/99
Person(s) interviewed: Tom's mother
Interviewer: Miss Sand (Action Team member)

Student Profile: What is the student good at or what are some strengths that the student brings to school?
Loving child, creative, lots of energy, athletic

Step 1A: Interview Teacher/Staff/Parent

Description of the Behavior

What does the problem behavior(s) look like? Says he doesn't know how to do homework. Talks back to mother and father, rips homework sheet, throws pencil down, cries, whines. **How often does the problem behavior(s) occur?** Every night that homework is expected. **How long does the problem behavior(s) last when it does occur?** Until dinner (about 2 hours). **How disruptive or dangerous is the problem behavior(s)?** Very frustrating for child and parents, big struggle, not dangerous.

Description of the Antecedent
Identifying Routines: When, where, and with whom are problem behaviors most likely?

Schedule (Times)	Activity	Specific Problem Behavior	Likelihood of Problem Behavior	With Whom Does Problem Occur?
7:15–7:45	Get up, get dressed	Doesn't like to get up—complains	Low High 1 ② 3 4 5 6	Mom
7:45–8:15	Breakfast		① 2 3 4 5 6	
8:15–8:30	Takes bus to school	Once or twice—peer argument	1 2 ③ 4 5 6	Peers
			1 2 3 4 5 6	
			1 2 3 4 5 6	
3:00–3:20	Takes bus home	Once or twice—peer argument	1 2 ③ 4 5 6	Peers
3:20–3:30	Snack		① 2 3 4 5 6	
3:30–?	Supposed to do homework	Refuses, crises, yells	1 2 3 4 5 ⑥	Mom and Dad
			1 2 3 4 5 6	

(continued)

FIGURE 3.7. Completed parent interview—Tom. The form itself is adapted by permission from March et al. (2000).

Summarize Antecedent (and Setting Events)

> **What situations seem to set off the problem behavior?** (difficult tasks, transitions, structured activities, small-group settings, teacher's request, particular individuals, etc.)
> After he's had snack and he's expected to start his homework.
>
> **When is the problem behavior most likely to occur?** (times of day and days of the week)
> At 3:30 every day that he has homework.
>
> **When is the problem behavior least likely to occur?** (times of day and days of the week)
> He doesn't have too much trouble getting up, going to school, or riding the bus.
>
> **Setting Events: Are there specific conditions, events, or activities that make the problem behavior worse?** (missed medication, history of academic failure, conflict at home, missed meals, lack of sleep, history of problems with peers, etc.)
> Behavior is worse if mother pushes him harder than usual to do the work. Behavior is worse on days when mother shows less patience with him.

Description of the Consequence

> **What usually happens after the behavior occurs?** (what is the teacher's reaction, how do other students react, is the student sent to the office, does the student get out of doing work, does the student get in a power struggle, etc.)
> Mother gets into argument with him. Mother is less able to pay attention to his younger siblings. Often he doesn't complete homework, so mother will sometimes do it for him so he doesn't get a failing grade at school.

- - - - - - End of Interview - - - - - -

Step 2A: Propose a Testable Explanation

Setting Event	Antecedent	Behavior	Consequence
Mother is in bad mood and has less patience	Expectation to do homework right after school	1. Cries, whines, yells, refuses to do work	Mother argues with him, sometimes does work for him
		2.	

Function of the Behavior

For each ABC sequence listed above, why do you think the behavior is occurring? (to get teacher attention, to get peer attention, gets desired object/activity, escapes undesirable activity, escapes demand, escapes particular people, etc.)

1. Tom is having the tantrums to get his mother's attention and to get out of doing work that he perceives as too hard.

How confident are you that your testable explanation is accurate?

Very sure		So-so			Not at all sure
6	5	④	3	2	1

FIGURE 3.7. *(continued)*

related concerns is to complete the interview form in relation to before-school and after-school routines. For example, *How does the student get home? Does she or he engage in problem behavior during transportation? What does the student do when she or he gets home? Is there a routine for homework?* An example of an F-BSP interview completed with the parents of Tom, is illustrated in Figure 3.7. This interview illustrates that problem behavior occurs most often at times when home-work completion is expected. The information gathered from the parents may help the Behavior Support Team initiate a collaborative home–school effort to en-courage Tom to consistently complete and turn in his homework.

Oftentimes, the student is not included in the FBA process. Recently, how-ever, research has demonstrated that students can contribute valuable informa-tion to a functional assessment of behavior. Reed et al. (1997) assessed the agreement between students and teachers regarding students' problem behav-iors. Teachers and students demonstrated high agreement on the predictors (77%), behaviors (85%), and consequences (77%), but much less agreement on the setting events that set up the problem behavior (26%). These results are sim-ilar to the pattern of results found by Nippe, Lewis-Palmer, and Sprague (1998). It is interesting to note that there was relatively low agreement between teachers and students on the setting events for problem behavior. This is not a surprising finding, since teachers may be unaware of many setting events that affect student behavior—for example, the student is irritable because he missed breakfast or is upset because of a family argument that occurred at home.

Students also identified more problem behaviors than did their teachers (Nippe et al., 1998; Reed et al., 1997). The differences in identified behaviors suggested that teachers reported on behaviors that were observable in the class-room, whereas students were able to include behaviors that occurred during transitions between classes or before and after school.

Teachers, parents, and other observers do not have access to the knowledge students possess regarding the occurrence, motivations, and context of their be-haviors. Clearly, students can contribute valuable information that might other-wise be missed in the FBA process. This information could be critical to the ef-fectiveness of intervention plans.

The F-BSP Protocol includes a student interview for identifying problem be-haviors, predictors, and consequences. The student interview is completed with the assistance of a member of the Action Team. (The Action Team is a subset of the Behavior Support Team.) Prior to interviewing the student, the Action Team member should fill in the student's daily schedule on the first page of the stu-dent interview. As the Action Team member conducts the interview, the student identifies the settings and times when she or he is most likely to get in trouble at school. In collaboration with the team member, the student then discusses what is occurring at these times to cause the misbehavior. Information gathered from the student interview can be used to generate hypothesis statements regarding

FUNCTIONAL BEHAVIORAL ASSESSMENT INTERVIEW—STUDENT

Student Name: Ronald _____ **Age:** 13 **Grade:** 7 **Date:** 2/7/99 _____

Interviewer: Mrs. Andrews (Action Team member) _____

Student Profile: What are the things you like to do, or do well, while at school? (activities, classes, helping others, etc.)

Likes hanging out with friends during lunch. Gym class is fun and is good at it. Science can be okay sometimes. Likes the school parties and dances

Step 1B: Interview Student

Description of the Behavior

> **What are some things you do that get you in trouble or that are a problem at school?** (talking out, not getting work done, fighting, etc.)
>
> "Fight with other kids. Punch other kids in the arm. Talk back to the teacher."
>
> **How often do you _____?** (Insert the behavior listed by the student)
>
> "I get in fights in social studies and science whenever we have to do that stupid group work. I think that's usually on Friday."
>
> "I don't talk back to the teachers too often. Just when they give us stupid, boring stuff to do."
>
> **How long does _____ usually last each time it happens?**
>
> "Fights last until the teacher notices. Then I get to leave and just go to the office for a while."
>
> **How serious is _____?** (Do you or another student end up getting hurt? Are other students distracted?)
>
> "I've ended up hurting some kids before, not too bad though"

Description of the Antecedent
Identifying Routines: When, where, and with whom are problem behaviors most likely?

Schedule (Times)	Activity	Specific Problem Behavior	Likelihood of Problem Behavior	With Whom Does Problem Occur?
			Low High	
8:20–9:15	Science	Fights	1 2 ③ 4 5 6	Peers
9:20–10:15	Math	Don't understand work	1 2 3 4 5 ⑥	Teacher
10:20–11:15	Reading	Don't understand work	1 2 3 4 5 ⑥	Teacher
11:20–12:15	Spanish	Don't understand work	1 2 3 ④ 5 6	Teacher
12:20–1:00	Lunch		① 2 3 4 5 6	
1:05–2:00	Social Studies	Fights	1 2 3 4 ⑤ 6	Peers
2:05–3:00	Physical Education		1 ② 3 4 5 6	
Other	Transitions between classrooms	Fights	1 2 3 4 5 ⑥	Peers
Other	Working with substitutes		1 2 ③ 4 5 6	Teacher
Other	Getting help		1 2 ③ 4 5 6	Teacher/Peers

(continued)

FIGURE 3.8. Completed student interview—Ronald. The form itself is adapted by permission from March et al. (2000).

Summarize Antecedent (and Setting Events)

What kind of things make it more likely that you will have this problem? (difficult tasks, transitions, structured activities, small-group settings, teacher's request, particular individuals, etc.) "Fighting? If I have to work with J. D. or M. L. because they always say something stupid to me. Especially if the teacher is working at his desk, so he's not watching us too good." **When and where is the problem most likely to happen?** (days of week, specific classes, hallways, bathrooms) "I get in the most fights in social studies, sometimes in science class too because we have to work in groups and J.D. is in that class." **When is the problem behavior least likely to occur?** (days of week, specific classes, hallways, bathrooms) "I never get in trouble in gym or lunch—that's fun time. Nobody bugs me to do anything." **Setting Events: Is there there anything that happens before or after school or in between classes that makes it more likely that you'll have a problem?** (missed medication, history of academic failure, conflict at home, missed meals, lack of sleep, history of problems with peers, etc.) "If I get into a fight with somebody on Monday, I might get into it with him again on Tuesday, 'cuz I'm still mad."

Description of the Consequence

What usually happens after the problem occurs? (what is the teacher's reaction, how do other students react, is the student sent to the office, does the student get out of doing work, does the student get in a power struggle, etc.) "Usually the other kid gets mad or hurt and leaves me alone. Then the teacher tells me to knock it off. He hardly ever yells at the other kids even if they started it. But I don't want to be there, so I just keep bugging them until he sends me out of the room."

- - - - - - End of Interview - - - - - -

Step 2B: Develop a Testable Explanation

Setting Event	Antecedent	Behavior	Consequence
Presence of J. D. or M. L., previous fight	Cooperative group work, not monitored, negative peer comment	1. Punch other students. Unable to work in group.	Classmate withdraws. Teacher reprimands. Eventually sent to office and escapes situation.
		2.	
		3.	

Function of the Behavior

For each ABC sequence listed above, why do you think the behavior is occurring? (to get teacher attention, to get peer attention, gets desired object/activity, escapes undesirable activity, escapes demand, escapes particular people, etc.)

1. Ronald is hitting other student to get out of an aversive situation. He wants to escape the negative peer comments that occur during cooperative group work.

FIGURE 3.8. (*continued*)

the function and predictors of the problem behavior. An example student interview for Ronald is illustrated in Figure 3.8. A blank copy of the student interview is included in Appendix B as part of the complete F-BSP Protocol.

Middle school and high school students have to travel from class to class, usually on an hourly basis. This means the students must make multiple transitions. Ronald reports engaging in problem behaviors during transition times on a frequent basis. The teacher was unaware of this information and did not report it during the teacher interview. Because transitions are often a time when problem behavior is likely to occur, it is very important to include them in the routine matrix of the student-guided interview.

After the student interview is completed, the Behavior Support Team analyzes the information to generate a testable hypothesis for when, where, why, and with whom the problem behavior is occurring. The testable hypothesis generated by the student interview can be compared to the testable hypotheses generated by the teacher (and parent) interview(s). The stronger the agreement between the two testable hypotheses, the more confident the team will be in the accuracy of their assessment. The F-BSP Protocol includes a section to compare the hypotheses between teacher and student interviews and to rerate the confidence in the testable hypothesis. This is illustrated in Figure 3.9.

We should point out that we have found it difficult to obtain FBA information from students in second grade or younger. Young children typically have less awareness of, and insight into, their behavior than do older children.

Observation

At least one observation of the student is necessary to complete the full FBA. Ideally, observations are conducted until a predictable pattern of behavior is observed. The student should be observed in the setting in which problem behaviors typically occur, as indicated by the teacher, parent, and student inter-

Step 3: Rate Your Confidence in the Testable Explanation

If you completed both interviews, was there agreement on these parts? (Y/N)
(a) Setting Events ___ (b) Antecedents Y___ (c) Behaviors Y/N (d) Consequences Y___ (e) Function Y___
Student focused on fewer problem behaviors than teacher
How confident are you that your testable explanation is accurate?

Very sure			So-so		Not at all sure
6	5	④	3	2	1

FIGURE 3.9. F-BSP Protocol, Step 3.

views. Multiple observation systems are available. The Behavior Support Team may choose to use any adequate observation system with which they are familiar. An adequate observation system will provide objective quantifiable data regarding the (1) antecedents of problem behavior, (2) occurrence of problem behavior, and (3) maintaining consequences of problem behavior. The Functional Assessment Observation (FAO) form is one useful tool for conducting functional observations of behavior. "The FAO indicates: a) the number of events of problem behavior, b) the problem behaviors that occur together, c) the times when problem behavior events are most and least likely to occur, d) events that predict problem behavior events, e) perceptions about the maintaining function of problem behaviors, and f) actual consequences following problem behavior events" (O'Neill et al., 1997, p. 37). If desired and feasible, multiple observations over several days can be recorded on one FAO sheet. A sample of a completed FAO for Vera is included in Figure 3.10. A blank copy of the FAO is included in Appendix H. Instructions for completion of this form can be obtained in the book *Functional Assessment and Program Development for Problem Behavior: A Practical Handbook* (O'Neill et al., 1997).

The purpose of this observation is to test the validity of the hypothesis statements and to resolve any discrepancies between the teacher-generated and the student-generated hypotheses. The FAO is completed by a member of the Behavior Support Team who has demonstrated competency conducting FBA observations. The sample FAO for Vera confirms the testable hypotheses about the predictors and maintaining consequences of Vera's problem behavior. The problem behavior reported in the interviews was the same type of problem behavior noted during the observation. Most of the problem behavior occurred during large-group activities. Most of the problem behavior was maintained by adult attention to the problem behavior and to get access to items she desires. The close correspondence between the interviews and the observations increases the team's confidence in the testable hypothesis, from which they will build the BSP for this student.

Often, it is useful to conduct a peer-referenced observation in addition to the FBA observation. The major purpose of the peer-referenced comparison observation is to determine the severity of the student's problem behavior relative to his or her same-age peers. The student's behavior is compared to the behavior of a composite of the student's classmates. The requisite data include percentage of time on-task, percentage of time off-task, and percentage of time engaged in problem behaviors. This observation typically lasts for 15–30 minutes. An example of one line of data from a sample Peer Comparison Observation Form is included in Figure 3.11. Summaries of observational data for Vera are included in Figure 3.12.

The summary of peer observation data clearly validates the teacher's con-

Functional Assessment Observation Form

Name: _Vera_   Starting Date: _1/15/99_   Ending Date: _1/17/99_

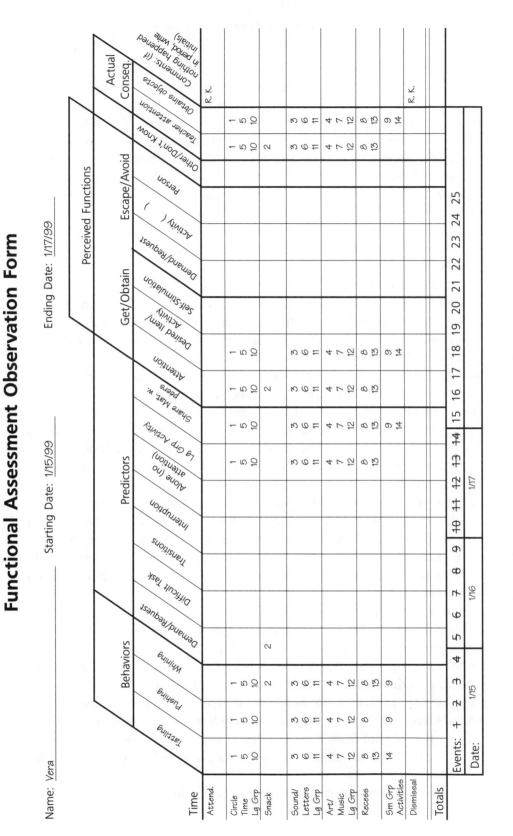

FIGURE 3.10. Functional Assessment Observation Form—Vera. The form itself is from O'Neill et al., *Functional Assessment for Problem Behavior: A Practical Handbook* (2nd ed.). © 1997. Adapted by permission of Wadsworth, an imprint of the Wadsworth Group, a division of Thomson Learning. Fax 800-730-2215.

52

Student: Vera   School: Wilson
Elem
Date: 1/15   Grade: Kinder
Setting: Classroom   Activity: Circle Tm.
Begin Time: 9:15   End Time: 9:35
Observer: Mr. Green

On = On task   Off = Off task
T = In appropriate talk   OS = Out of seat
F = Fidgeting
Beh 2 = Tattling
Beh 2 = Pushing

	:10		:20		:30		:40		:50		:00
(Stdt)	T F	(On)	T F	(On)	(T) F	On	T F	On	T F	On	T F	(On)
Peer	OS	Off	OS	Off	OS	(Off)	OS	(Off)	(OS)	(Off)	OS	Off
M F	Beh 2		Beh 2		(Beh 2)		Beh 2		Beh 2		Beh 2	
	Beh 2		Beh 2		Beh 2		(Beh 2)		Beh 2		Beh 2	

	:10		:20		:30		:40		:50		:00
Stdt	T F	(On)	T F	(On)	T F	(On)	T F	(On)	(T) F	On	T F	On
(Peer)	OS	Off	OS	Off	OS	Off	OS	Off	OS	(Off)	(OS)	(Off)
M (F)	Beh 2		Beh 2		Beh 2		Beh 2		Beh 2		Beh 2	
	Beh 2		Beh 2		Beh 2		Beh 2		Beh 2		Beh 2	

FIGURE 3.11. Sample line of data from Peer Comparison Observation Form.

cerns that Vera's behavior is significantly discrepant from her peers and is disruptive to the classroom. She is off-task 30% of the time and she engages in tattling behavior that distracts the teacher from instruction during 12% of the intervals. This is compared to her peers, who are only off-task 17% of the time and engaged in tattling behavior during 0% of intervals observed.

After completing the additional interviews and at least one observation, the Behavior Support Team has collected enough information to verify or modify the original testable hypothesis. At this point, they are ready to design a BSP and form an Action Plan. The following chapter outlines how the Behavior Support Team develops a function-based BSP.

January 15: 9:15–9:35 (Classroom—Circle Time)		
	Student	Peer comparison
On-task	70%	83%
Off-task	30%	17%
Talk-outs	6%	3%
Out of seat	0%	0%
Fidgeting	0%	0%
Tattling	12%	0%
Pushing	0%	0%

FIGURE 3.12. Sample summary of data from Peer Comparison Observation Form.

SUPPLEMENTARY SECTION

References on Functional Analysis

- Carr, E. G., Yarbrough, S. C., & Langdon, N. A. (1997). Effects of idiosyncratic stimulus variables on functional analysis outcomes. *Journal of Applied Behavior Analysis*, *30*(4), 673–686.
- Daly, E. J., III, Witt, J. C., Martens, B. K., & Dool, E. J. (1997). A model for conducting a functional analysis of academic performance problems. *School Psychology Review*, *26*(4), 554–574.
- Derby, K. M., Wacker, D. P., Peck, S., Sasso, G., DeRaad, A., Berg, W., Asmus, J., & Ulrich, S. (1994). Functional analysis of separate topographies of aberrant behavior. *Journal of Applied Behavior Analysis*, *27*(2), 267–278.
- Harding, J., Wacker, D., Cooper, L., Millard, T., & Jensen-Kovalan, P. (1994). Brief hierarchical assessment of potential treatment components with children in an outpatient clinic. *Journal of Applied Behavior Analysis*, *27*(2), 291–300.
- Haynes, S. N. (1998). The assessment–treatment relationship and functional analysis in behavior therapy. *European Journal of Psychological Assessment*, *14*(1), 26–35.
- Haynes, S. N., Leisen, M. B., & Blaine, D. D. (1997). Design of individualized behavioral treatment programs using functional analytic clinical case models. *Psychological Assessment*, *9*(4), 334–348.
- Kahng, S. W., & Iwata, B. A. (1999). Correspondence between outcomes of brief and extended functional analyses. *Journal of Applied Behavior Analysis*, *32*, 149–159.
- Meyer, K. A. (1999). Functional analysis and treatment of problem behavior exhibited by elementary school children. *Journal of Applied Behavior Analysis*, *32*, 229–232.
- Northup, J., Wacker, D., Sasso, G., Steege, M., Cigrand, K., Cook, J., & DeRaad, A. (1991). A brief functional analysis of aggressive and alternative behavior in an outclinic setting. *Journal of Applied Behavior Analysis*, *24*(3), 509–522.
- Selinske, J. E., Greer, R., & Lodhi, S. (1991). A functional analysis of the comprehensive application of behavior analysis to schooling. *Journal of Applied Behavior Analysis*, *24*(1), 107–117.
- Vollmer, T. R., Iwata, B. A., Duncan, B. A., & Lerman, D. C. (1993). Extensions of multielement functional analyses using reversal-type designs. *Journal of Developmental and Physical Disabilities*, *5*(4), 311–325.
- Vollmer, T. R., Marcus, B. A., Ringdahl, J. E., & Roane, H. S. (1995). Progressing from brief assessments to extended experimental analyses in the evaluation of aberrant behavior. *Journal of Applied Behavior Analysis*, *28*(4), 561–576.
- Wacker, D. P., Steege, M., & Berg, W. K. (1988). Use of single-case designs to evaluate manipulable influences on school performance. *School Psychology Review*, *17*(4), 651–657.
- Watson, T. S., Ray, K. P., Turner, H. S., & Logan, P. (1999). Teacher-implemented functional analysis and treatment: A method for linking assessment to intervention. *School Psychology Review*, *28*, 292–302.

CHAPTER 4

Designing a Behavior Support Plan

INTRODUCTION

Using the three case examples introduced in Chapter 3, this chapter will demonstrate how to use a FBA to design a BSP. A BSP is a written record that summarizes the FBA information and documents the intervention plan. An effective BSP describes in detail how, by whom, and in what situations the intervention strategies will be implemented. In addition, an effective BSP should include monitoring and evaluation procedures.

COMPETING BEHAVIORS

The first step in designing a BSP is to generate strategies for *reducing problem behaviors* and *increasing appropriate, replacement behaviors*. By ensuring that the intervention is linked with the FBA, the efficiency, efficacy, and relevance of the BSP are increased. The Competing Behavior Pathway form is one instrument used to create a link between the FBA and the BSP. The Competing Behavior Pathway form is incorporated into the F-BSP Protocol. A blank copy is included in Appendix B (Step 6: Build a Competing Behavior Pathway).

Competing behaviors are behaviors that are mutually exclusive. An individual cannot simultaneously engage in two competing behaviors. For example, running and walking are competing behaviors. Applied to BSPs, problem behaviors and desired behaviors are competing behaviors. A child cannot simultaneously engage in "ignore the teacher" and "follow directions."

The purpose of the Competing Behavior Pathway step is threefold: (1) to highlight the importance of building the behavior support plan around the hypothesis statement; (2) to identify competing behavioral alternatives (desired or acceptable behaviors) to the problem behavior; and (3) to determine strategies for making the problem behavior ineffective, inefficient, or irrelevant through changes to the routine or environment.

The Behavior Support Team uses the Competing Behavior Pathway step to brainstorm multiple strategies for changing the routine by (1) modifying the predictors that set off the problem behavior; (2) teaching appropriate or alternate behaviors; and (3) modifying ineffective consequences that have maintained rather than eliminated the problem behavior. The intervention strategies developed by referring to the Competing Behavior Pathway step will become the basis of the behavior support plan.

To clarify, examine the sample Competing Behavior Pathway form for Tom in Figure 4.1. The middle section of the Competing Behaviors Pathway form restates the hypothesis statement. Put simply, *"This is what is happening now."* The top section identifies the appropriate, desired behavior expected of the child: *"This is what we'd like to have happen eventually."* The bottom section indicates alternative behaviors that serve the same function as the problem behavior, but are more acceptable to the teacher, other school staff, and parents: *"This is what we'd be happy with in the meantime."* Often, it is not the function of the problem behavior that is offensive (e.g., to receive adult attention). Rather, it is the strategies the child uses to achieve that function (e.g., causing serious disruptions in the class) that is problematic. To create an effective BSP, the Behavior Support Team and referring teacher must teach the child alternative, acceptable behaviors that serve the same function as the problem behavior (e.g., teaching the child to request help for difficult tasks).

Consider the case example of Tom by referring to Figure 4.1. Tom's primary problem behavior was *"refusing to do work and causing disruption."* The function of his problem behavior was *"gaining teacher and peer attention."* A desired alternative (i.e., competing behavior) could be *"completing work without disruption."* An acceptable alternative behavior, serving the same function as the problem behavior while also competing with the problem behavior, could be *"requesting intermittent attention and assistance from the teacher or a competent peer."* If the student begins to consistently engage in the acceptable alternative, this alternative will serve as a stepping-stone to the "desired behavior." For example, Tom's teachers and parents would like him to eventually be able to work independently without overreliance on his teacher or peers. The Competing Behavior Pathway forms for Vera and Ronald are presented in Figures 4.2 and 4.3.

Once the team has determined the desired behavior and an acceptable alternative to the problem behavior, they must generate strategies to facilitate the student's performance of these behaviors. In order to make the problem behavior ineffective, inefficient, and irrelevant, the team should focus on strategies

Step 6: Build a Competing Behavior Pathway

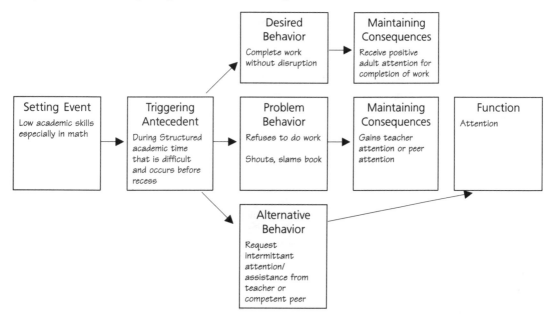

Setting Event Strategies	Antecedent Strategies	Behavior Teaching Strategies	Consequence Strategies
Assess if math curriculum is at appropriate level Additional instruction in math 1:1 instruction in math	Define expectations Divide one long recess into two short recesses that occur earlier Precorrect Move desk to quiet area	Teach expectations Teach about reward system Teach to ask for help through role play	Reward expectations Ignore inappropriate behavior Earn "attention tickets" Earn other tangibles—e.g., art supplies or time to work on art projects.

FIGURE 4.1. Behavior Support Plan, Step 6—Tom. The form itselft is from O'Neill et al., *Functional Assessment for Problem Behavior: A Practical Handbook* (2nd ed.). © 1997. Adapted by permission of Wadsworth, an imprint of the Wadsworth Group, a division of Thomson Learning. Fax 800-730-2215.

Step 6: Build a Competing Behavior Pathway

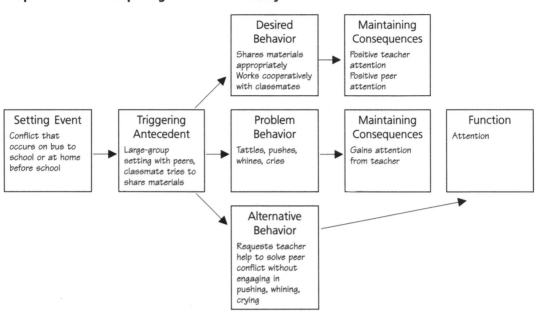

Setting Event Strategies	Antecedent Strategies	Behavior Teaching Strategies	Consequence Strategies
Increase communication between home and school	Define expectations	Teach expectations	Reward expectations
	Precorrect	Teach to request help	Give positive attention for working appropriately and cooperating
Increase communication between bus and school	Increase number of supplies available	Teach to problem solve with peers	
	Seat next to competent peer	Teach to take turns using materials	Reward system to earn rewards for entire group
	Pair with peer who is a good role model		

FIGURE 4.2. Behavior Support Plan, Step 6—Vera. The form itselft is from O'Neill et al., *Functional Assessment for Problem Behavior: A Practical Handbook* (2nd ed.). © 1997. Adapted by permission of Wadsworth, an imprint of the Wadsworth Group, a division of Thomson Learning. Fax 800-730-2215.

Step 6: Build a Competing Behavior Pathway

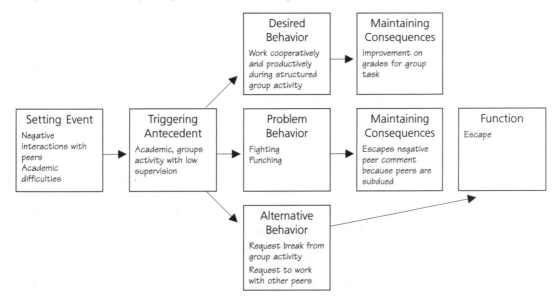

		Desired Behavior	Maintaining Consequences
		Work cooperatively and productively during structured group activity	Improvement on grades for group task

Setting Event	Triggering Antecedent	Problem Behavior	Maintaining Consequences	Function
Negative interactions with peers Academic difficulties	Academic, groups activity with low supervision	Fighting Punching	Escapes negative peer comment because peers are subdued	Escape

Alternative Behavior
Request break from group activity
Request to work with other peers

Setting Event Strategies	Antecedent Strategies	Behavior Teaching Strategies	Consequence Strategies
Physically separate from peers with whom he has the most negative interactions Assess academic Skills Individualize/modify curriculum to match skills	Define expectations Reduce number of group activities expected Allow choice of group or individual projects Increase his monitoring/ supervision Check-in system Pair with peer who provides good role model	Teach expectations Teach Ronald to request a break or change in partners Teach problem-solving skills	Reward expectattions Emphasize connections between actions and grades Reward Ronald for appropriate behavior

FIGURE 4.3. Behavior Support Plan, Step 6—Ronald. The form itselft is from O'Neill et al., *Functional Assessment for Problem Behavior: A Practical Handbook* (2nd ed.). © 1997. Adapted by permission of Wadsworth, an imprint of the Wadsworth Group, a division of Thomson Learning. Fax 800-730-2215.

that teach the child new skills and behaviors or that alter aspects of the child's routine. At each point in the hypothesis statement (setting event, triggering antecedent, problem behavior, consequence), adults can alter the student's routine to improve the likelihood that the child will be successful—that problem behavior will be decreased and appropriate behavior will be increased. The Competing Behavior Pathway form (Step 6 of the F-BSP Protocol) provides space to brainstorm strategies for (1) setting event manipulations, (2) triggering antecedent manipulations, (3) behavioral teaching, and (4) consequence manipulations. The following are some strategies suggested on Ronald's Competing Behavior Pathway form (Figure 4.3): (1) to change the setting event—*physically separate Ronald from those peers with whom he has the most negative interactions*; (2) to change the antecedents—*allow Ronald a choice of group or individual projects or increase his monitoring/supervision*; (3) to teach new behaviors—*teach Ronald to request a break or a change in partners*; (4) to change the consequences—*reward Ronald for appropriate behavior*.

At this point in designing the BSP, the Behavior Support Team is brainstorming. Team members should not censor any suggestions. Later the team will consider the list of ideas and decide which strategies fit best within the contextual limitations of the school and classroom. By brainstorming, the team creates a "bank" of ideas from which to draw. The team may choose a few strategies to begin with and then find that the original plan does not work for a particular child. The team will find that modifying an ineffective BSP is much easier when there are a multitude of additional options to go back to and choose from.

The primary reasons for using the Competing Behavior Pathway and for including parents and teachers in the development of the BSP are: "1) it increases the link between intervention procedures and functional assessment results; 2) it increases the fit between the values, skills, resources, and routines of the people who will carry out the plan and the procedures that will be employed; 3) it increases the logical coherence among the different procedures that could be used in a multi-element plan of support; and 4) it increases the fidelity with which the plan is ultimately implemented" (O'Neill et al., 1997, p. 69).

CONTEXTUAL FIT

A second, important consideration in designing a BSP is to increase the fit between the behavior support plan and the values, skills, resources, and routines of the people who will carry out the plan. This concept is called *contextual* fit. The importance of contextual fit cannot be overstated. Imagine designing the "perfect" BSP, one that if implemented properly could not fail to work, only to find that it *cannot* be implemented properly. The Behavior Support Team may find that they have forgotten to consider important practical constraints such as time, resources, finances, skills, facilities issues, attitudes, or beliefs.

The importance of contextual fit can be illustrated with a few examples.

Example 1

The Behavior Support Team may choose to incorporate a home–school note into Ronald's BSP. First, the team identifies a behavioral goal for each class period. On a daily basis, Ronald checks in with each teacher to mark if he has met his goal during that class period. At the end of the day he checks out with the school counselor and takes the behavior sheet home. His parents are expected to review the behavior sheet, sign it, write an encouraging comment for Ronald, and return it to the school.

This is a sound strategy, one that has been demonstrated to work with middle school students at risk for serious behavior problems. Parents could be taught to understand and participate in the system. *However, what if Ronald's parents are illiterate?* In this case, they will not be able to read the daily report or add comments to it. *How will this affect Ronald's success? Will it embarrass the parents and alienate them from the school?* These types of problems can be easily avoided (once contextual fit is considered) with slight modifications. For example, the school could make phone contact rather than paper contact with the student's parents.

Example 2

Part of Tom's original BSP involved increasing communication between his homeroom teacher and his resource room teacher. Tom's resource room teacher would write a note about his behavior during class and Tom would carry the note back with him to his homeroom teacher. Two problems arose: (1) When Tom is angry (e.g., if he receives a negative report on his behavior) he has a tendency to rip his papers into shreds; and (2) Tom is very forgetful and distractible and often forgets or loses the resource room teacher's note. The intervention strategy does not have to be eliminated. Rather, by considering contextual fit, the strategy could be modified and made more effective. To eliminate the first problem, the behavior note could be laminated and reused, using a grease pencil, on a daily basis. To eliminate the second problem, the responsibility for sending the note between teachers could be placed on the teachers, not on the student. Another possible solution would be to reward Tom for delivering the note to his homeroom teacher, whether or not the note contained good news or bad news.

Often, problems of contextual fit revolve around issues of time and effort.

The team may design a comprehensive BSP that requires more time and effort than the teacher has to give. In designing BSPs, the Behavior Support Team should emphasize effectiveness *and* efficiency. For example, rather than design a BSP that requires constant teacher monitoring and interaction, the Behavior Support Team might create a BSP that includes self-management or self-monitoring strategies by the student. By taking some of the burden off the teacher, while teaching the child responsibility and independence, a BSP that includes self-management achieves a double purpose.

INDIVIDUALIZING THE BEHAVIOR SUPPORT PLAN

One of the most difficult challenges in intervening with children with behavior problems is their variability in response to treatment. Intervention strategies may be effective for some children but not for others, or may only be effective for certain children in certain settings. When a BSP does not incorporate FBA, different children exhibiting the same type of behavior problems may receive the same intervention, even if the problem behavior serves different functions for different children.

Imagine a second-grade student who frequently causes serious disruption in the classroom. Based on an FBA, the following hypothesis statement is generated: *"After the teacher gives Reuben a difficult reading assignment, Reuben crumples his paper and starts flinging spit wads at his peers in order to get out of the assignment."* An FBA of the same behavior exhibited by a different child yields a slightly different hypothesis statement. For example, *"When Rita is in reading class and she has not received any individual teacher attention for over 10 minutes, she starts crumpling her assignment and flinging spit wads at her classmates in order to get the teacher's attention."* The behavior of the two students looks exactly the same. However, the predictors and function of the behavior are quite different and suggest very different BSPs.

Assume that the teacher employs a very common response to disruptive behavior: each time a child causes a serious disruption he or she is made to sit in the hallway for 10 minutes. This generic approach to managing problem behavior is actually rewarding to Reuben! By being placed in the hallway he obtains what he is seeking: escape from his reading assignment. Placing the student in the hallway might be a more effective discipline strategy for Rita. This strategy further reduces the amount of teacher attention Rita receives. In the future, she is less likely to try that strategy to obtain teacher attention.

A function-based approach considers the unique features of the situation, the child, or the behavior that predict the success or failure of a behavioral intervention. Use of FBA procedures helps the Behavior Support Team to design behavior support plans for each student with whom they work.

A second important consideration in individualizing BSPs is the choice of re-inforcers. Many BSPs will incorporate a reward system to reinforce the child's appropriate behavior. The choice of reinforcers should be based on what is motivating to this *particular* student, not based on what an adult believes is motivating to *all* students. For example, in Tom's original BSP, the team decided that he could earn 5 minutes of computer time if he exhibited appropriate behavior during typically problematic routines. The plan was implemented, but Tom's behavior got worse. *Why did Tom's behavior get worse after implementing the intervention?* The team was perplexed until they spoke with Tom. After speaking with Tom, they discovered that his least favorite activity was using the computer! In effect, the team was "rewarding" Tom's good behavior with an activity that was actually punishing to him. Upon further questioning, the team learned that Tom enjoys using art supplies. The BSP was modified so that Tom could earn 5 minutes of art time instead of computer time. Immediately, his behavior improved as he worked toward a personally meaningful reinforcer. Information about a student's preferred activities and reinforcers can be easily obtained through the student-guided interview, as described in Chapter 3.

DOCUMENTING A BEHAVIOR SUPPORT PLAN

After completing the Competing Behavior Pathway form and deciding which strategies will be used, the Behavior Support Team documents these decisions in the form of a written BSP. Each school district typically provides their own forms for documenting BSPs. A sample form for each of the three case examples is presented in Figures 4.4, 4.5, and 4.6. A blank copy of this form is incorporated into the F-BSP Protocol (see Appendix B, Step 7: Selection Intervention Strategies).

The team chooses among the strategies generated on the Competing Behavior Pathway form and lists each strategy on the BSP (this is Step 7: Select Intervention Strategies on the F-BSP Protocol). At times, the team may add strategies that were not used in Step 6. It is critical to document who is responsible for implementing the strategy, when it will be implemented, and how it will be implemented. If the student is to be taught a new behavior, the plan must indicate who will teach the child the behavior. Someone on the team should be designated to discuss the BSP with the student. This critical step is often forgotten or neglected. If the BSP is to be effective, the student *must* be informed about its expectations, goals, and rewards, and must have the opportunity to ask questions about the plan.

An essential component of the BSP is documenting a plan for managing inappropriate behavior. The child's inappropriate behavior has been built over a long period of time. It may take an equally long period of time to replace the inappropriate behavior with appropriate behavior. The adults in the student's rou-

Step 7: Select Intervention Strategies

Tasks	Person Responsible	By When	Review Date	Evaluation Decision • Monitor • Modify • Discontinue
1. Math assessment and curriculum individualization	Math resource teacher	Two weeks— 11/1/99	2–3 weeks 11/8/99	
2. Role-play how to make appropriate requests for help	School psychologist	By 10/25/99	11/8/99	
3. Allow Tom to earn "coupons" to trade in at school store or for 5 minutes of art time as a reward for appropriate behavior throughout a class period	Teacher	Begin 10/22/99	11/8/99	
4. Design behavior card and "coupons." Communicate to all relevant adults how the behavior card will be used	School psychologist	10/21/99	11/8/99	
5. Explain behavior support plan to student	Teacher	10/21/99	11/8/99	

*If emergency behavior management procedures are necessary, attach crisis plan as separate sheet.

FIGURE 4.4. Behavior Support Plan, Step 7—Tom.

Step 7: Select Intervention Strategies

Tasks	Person Responsible	By When	Review Date	Evaluation Decision • Monitor • Modify • Discontinue
1. "1-minute check-in." Teacher provides positive attention first thing in the morning by asking Vera how her morning was and by precorrecting her about behavioral expectations for school	Kindergarten teacher	Next Tuesday 1/25/99	Within 2– 3 weeks 2/6/99	
2. Practice role playing with student the right way to share with other students and how to ask for help from teacher rather than tattle	Kindergarten teacher	1/28/99	2/6/99	
3. Provide positive attention (smile, encouragement, pat on back) after every 10 minutes of cooperative, nondisruptive work exhibited by Vera	Kindergarten teacher	1/25/99	2/6/99	
4. Explain behavior support plan to Vera	School psychologist	Day before it starts 1/24/99	2/6/99	
5. Ignore tattling behavior	Kindergarten teacher	1/25/99	2/6/99	

*If emergency behavior management procedures are necessary, attach crisis plan as separate sheet.

FIGURE 4.5. Behavior Support Plan, Step 7—Vera.

Step 7: Select Intervention Strategies

Tasks	Person Responsible	By When	Review Date	Evaluation Decision • Monitor • Modify • Discontinue
1. Provide student with choice to complete project individually or with group	Science and social studies teachers	Next day 2/11/99	2–3 weeks 2/28/99	
2. Increase supervision of group activities	Teachers	2/11/99	2/28/99	
3. Student participate in peer conflict resolution group	Led by school counselor	Ongoing group: begin 2/18/99	2/28/99	
4. Student participate in relaxation skills group	Led by school counselor	Ongoing group: begin 2/19/99	2/28/99	
5. Teach student to request a break from work or to request a change in work partners	School psychologist	2/11/99	2/28/99	
6. Respond to student requests for break and praise student for appropriate use of the strategy	Teachers	2/11/99	2/28/99	
7. Create behavior card for monitoring behavior in class	School psychologist	2/11/99	2/28/99	
8. Explain behavior support plan to student	School psychologist	2/11/99	2/28/99	

*If emergency behavior management procedures are necessary, attach crisis plan as separate sheet.

FIGURE 4.6. Behavior Support Plan, Step 7—Ronald.

tines should have a consistent plan for responding to inappropriate behavior. In the case of mild misbehavior, the plan may be simply to ignore the behavior. Severe or dangerous behavior may require a crisis plan.

A crisis plan was developed for responding to Ronald's severely disruptive or dangerous behavior. This crisis plan, as presented in Table 4.1, should be attached to the BSP. The crisis plan should be based on data collected during the FBA and during discussion of the school's resources and the staff's availability to assist each other. Each of the staff involved in Ronald's plan agreed to their part in the plan. A copy of the crisis plan is distributed to the principal and each of Ronald's teachers.

Perhaps the most important step in documenting the BSP is to obtain the written agreement of everyone involved in the implementation of the plan, including the student, teacher, parent/guardian, and other members of the Action Team. Finally, the team should specify a date when the plan will be reviewed, evaluated, and modified if necessary. A copy of the BSP should be provided to each of the student's teachers and to the student's parents. A copy should also be kept on file in the Behavior Support Team's records.

Designing an effective BSP is both a science and an art. To be effective, each BSP needs to address numerous critical features that have been discussed in this book. Some of these critical features include (1) an observable, measurable description of the problem behavior; (2) a testable explanation regarding the function of the problem behavior; (3) strategies for extinguishing problem behavior; (4) strategies for reinforcing appropriate behavior; (5) strategies for measuring and evaluating behavioral change; and (6) consideration of contextual fit. Although Step 7 of the F-BSP Protocol lists the actual strategies that will be employed, the entire document, Steps 1–8, can be considered part of the final BSP. The F-BSP Protocol includes all of the critical features of a good, function-based BSP without creating redundancy by requiring the same information on multiple forms (e.g., on the Interview form, the BSP form, the Evaluation form, etc.). Hor-

---

TABLE 4.1. Sample Crisis Plan for Ronald

1. Be aware of cues that student is upset.
2. Try to calm student. Separate student from peers if possible.
3. If problem gets worse, notify school principal.
4. School counselor will cover gym teacher's class
5. Gym teacher will come to talk with student and escort him to gym.
6. Student takes a 10-minute time-out outside of gym.
7. Student is verbally praised for calming himself and for taking time-out appropriately.
8. The gym teacher reminds student of expectations upon returning to class.
9. The gym teacher (or other adult) escorts student back to class.

ner et al. (1999–2000) designed a checklist for assessing the quality of BSPs. This checklist is reproduced in Figure 4.7; a copy of the checklist is also included in Appendix I.

Although a complete treatment of the subject of designing BSP is beyond the scope of this chapter, the reader can refer to the Supplementary Section of this chapter for a list of resources on this topic.

SUPPLEMENTARY SECTION

Behavior Support Plans

- Artesani, A. J., & Mallar, L. (1998). Positive behavior supports in general education settings: Combining person-centered planning and functional analysis. *Intervention in School and Clinic, 34,* 33–38.
- Fad, K. M., Patton, J. R., & Polloway, E. A. (1998). *Behavioral intervention planning.* Austin, Texas: Pro-Ed.
- Horner, R. H., Sugai, G., Todd, A. W., & Lewis-Palmer, T. (1999–2000). Elements of behavior support plans: A technical brief. *Exceptionality, 8*(3), 205–215.
- Muscott, H. S. (1996). *Planning and implementing effective programs for school-aged children and youth with emotional/behavioral disorders within inclusive schools.* Mini-Library Series on Emotional/Behavioral Disorders. Council for Children with Behavioral Disorders.
- Repp, A. C., & Horner, R. H. (Eds.). (1999). *Functional analysis of problem behavior: From effective assessment to effective support.* Belmont, CA : Wadsworth.
- Sugai, G., Lewis-Palmer, T., & Hagan, S. (1998). Using functional assessments to develop behavior support plans. *Preventing School Failure, 43,* 6–13.

A CHECKLIST FOR ASSESSING THE QUALITY OF BEHAVIOR SUPPORT PLANNING: DOES THE PLAN (OR PLANNING PROCESS) HAVE THESE FEATURES?

When developing and implementing behavior support plans, judge the degree to which each of the following has been considered:

G = Good   O = Okay   P = Poor   N = Not applicable

1. ____ Define academic and lifestyle *context* for behavior support
2. ____ Operational description of problem behaviors
3. ____ Problem *routines* identified
4. ____ Functional assessment hypotheses stated
5. Intervention/*Foundations* (issues that cut across routines)
   a) ____ health and physiology
   b) ____ communication
   c) ____ mobility
   d) ____ predictability
   e) ____ control/choice
   f) ____ social relationships
   g) ____ activity patterns

6. Intervention/*Prevention* (make problem behavior irrelevant)
   a) ____ schedule
   b) ____ curriculum
   c) ____ instructional procedures

7. Intervention/*Teaching* (make problem behavior inefficient)
   a) ____ replacement skills
   b) ____ new adaptive skills

8. Intervention/*Consequences*
   Extinction (make problem behavior ineffective)
   a) ____ minimize positive reinforcement
   b) ____ minimize negative reinforcement
   Reinforcement (make appropriate behavior more effective)
   a) ____ maximize positive reinforcement
   Punishment (if needed)
   a) ____ negative consequences contingent upon problem behavior
   Safety/Emergency Intervention Plan
   a) ____ clear plan for what to do if/when problem behaviors occur

9. Evaluation and Assessment
   a) ____ define the information to be collected
   b) ____ define the measurement process
   c) ____ define decision-making process.

10. Ensure Contextual Fit
    a) ____ values
    b) ____ skills
    c) ____ resources
    d) ____ administrative system
    e) ____ perceptions that program is in best interest of student

FIGURE 4.7. Behavior support plan checklist. Adapted from Horner, Sugai, Todd, & Lewis-Palmer (1999–2000). Copyright 1999–2000 by Lawrence Erlbaum Associates. Adapted by permission.

CHAPTER 5

Evaluating and Modifying
the Behavior Support Plan

INTRODUCTION

This chapter demonstrates how to evaluate the effectiveness and feasibility of BSPs. The case examples presented in Chapter 3 will be used to illustrate strategies for evaluating and modifying the BSP.

Evaluation activities are essential elements of any effective BSP and must be integrated into the initial design of the plan. The critical elements of evaluation should (1) assess changes in behavior, (2) assess feasibility and acceptability of the BSP, and (3) assess student, parent, and teacher satisfaction. Evaluation procedures should be simple and efficient. The Behavior Support Team should collect sufficient data to make data-based decisions, without accumulating superfluous information. Additionally, the team should give careful consideration to issues of contextual fit. Evaluations should conclude with a plan to maintain behavioral gains over time.

RATIONALE

Of the steps involved in the assessment of and intervention for behavior problems, evaluation is the one step that is most likely to be ignored. Yet it is a critical part of embedding an effective program of individual behavioral support within a school. Without systematic evaluation, there are no objective means by which to determine if an intervention has been successful or if the efforts of the Behavior Support Team have been worthwhile. In an environment of scarce resources, a program that cannot provide evidence demonstrating that it is effective and worthwhile may be quickly abandoned or replaced. At the same time, an evaluation plan that is cumbersome or time-intensive will be discarded before its usefulness is tested. The Behavior Support Team should strive to make data-based decisions regarding whether to continue, monitor, or modify BSPs, using information that is simple and time-efficient to collect.

A well-planned evaluation can pinpoint problem areas in an unsuccessful intervention. Careful monitoring allows the team to identify problems early in the intervention process. For example, Ronald's home–school check-in system initially did not impact his behavior. He continued to engage in fights with fellow students with the same frequency and intensity as prior to the implementation of the BSP. The Behavior Support Team was ready to eliminate this strategy from Ronald's BSP. But after examining the daily data sheets, however, the team discovered that the home–school check-in system had not been fully implemented. Ronald's parents were not participating. Further examination of the problem revealed an issue of contextual fit. Both of Ronald's parents were functionally illiterate. They were not actively participating because they were *unable* to participate. Based on this knowledge, the Behavior Support Team modified the BSP to include regular phone contact rather than written contact between the school and Ronald's parents. This minor change resulted in increased participation by the parents and a concomitant improvement in Ronald's behavior.

Systematic evaluation enables the Behavior Support Team to make objective, data-based decisions. Routine presentation of individual data serves to update each member of the Action Team regarding the student's progress or lack thereof. Often, a student will make significant progress, yet still remain outside the limits of expected behavior. Without data, the team is likely to notice the student's continuing deviation from peers rather than improvements between his initial and his current behavior. The team may become discouraged, erroneously believing that their efforts did not make a difference. Routinely collected behavioral data can illustrate the student's improvement over time, encouraging and sustaining the team to keep up their efforts.

CRITICAL ELEMENTS

Problem behavior affects multiple people—the teacher, the principal, parents, students—each with their own unique assessment of and reaction to the problem behavior. Consequently, it is critical to collect multiple sets of evaluation data from multiple individuals. These different sources of information are discussed below.

Any person involved in the assessment and intervention can contribute to the evaluation, including the teacher, a parent, the student him- or herself, or other Action Team members. Involving the student in self-evaluation is a particularly useful strategy. Self-evaluation increases the salience of the student's own behavior to the student, often motivating and encouraging him or her to try harder. This phenomenon is also true for teachers. Teachers often remark that evaluation data are more meaningful if they themselves are personally involved in the evaluation.

Assessing Changes in Behavior

Numerous methods can be used to evaluate the impact of a BSP on reducing inappropriate behavior and increasing desired behavior. Frequency counts, individualized behavior rating scales, and observation are some of the most commonly used methods.

Frequency Count

One of the simplest evaluation methods is the frequency count. Teachers need an efficient strategy to record how often a child engages in a high-frequency problem behavior. Vera, for example, engages in tattling behavior multiple times per day, every day. Requiring the teacher to document Vera's tattling behavior after each occurrence could become burdensome and could also negatively impact instructional time. Much simpler means, for example, the "paperclip transfer strategy," could accomplish the same goal.

To use the paperclip transfer strategy, the teacher starts each day with a handful of paperclips (or other tiny objects) in one pocket. Each time the student engages in the problem behavior, the teacher transfers one paperclip to the opposite pocket. At the end of the day, the teacher counts how many paperclips have been transferred to the second pocket. The number of paperclips in the second pocket equals the incidence of problem behaviors (e.g., the number of times Vera tattled on another student) observed by the teacher. This number is recorded on a summary sheet. Progress or decline can be determined with a quick glance.

The summary sheet should be kept in a place that is easy to find and easy to remember. A very simple solution is to place a Post-it note in the teacher's lesson plan book (or any other place that is consistently used by the teacher on a daily basis). The summary Post-it would include one column for the date and one column for the number of behavioral incidents (see Figure 5.1). At the end of each week, the teacher would give the Post-it note to a designated member of the Action Team for more permanent recording of the weekly data.

Date	Number of times student tattled
2/2	√√√√
2/3	√√√

FIGURE 5.1. Summary of frequency data using a simple Post-it.

Behavior Rating Scale

A second evaluation method is to complete an individualized behavior rating scale on a regularly scheduled (hourly, daily, weekly) basis. First, the target behaviors are chosen and written on the summary sheet. Target behaviors can be problem behaviors (expect a decrease in frequency over time) or desired behaviors (expect an increase in frequency over time). Each target behavior is rated on a Likert scale, e.g., 0 = behavior did not occur; 1 = behavior occurred on a few occasions; 2 = behavior occurred frequently. For a younger child, the scale could be simplified to two items, e.g., yes = behavior occurred; no = behavior did not occur. Pictures of happy and sad faces could be substituted for a very young child or for a child with limited literacy skill. A sample of an individual behavior rating scale is illustrated in Figure 5.2.

Ratings are a means of providing feedback to a student about his or her behavior. Ratings also provide the teacher with regular opportunities to praise or reward the student for demonstrating appropriate behavior. Ratings that are made frequently (e.g., after each class period) are likely to have a stronger impact on the student's behavior than infrequent ratings. Ratings are most often made by the student or by the teacher, rather than by an outside observer. Ratings made by the student are incorporated into a self-management behavioral intervention.

The team must decide how frequently ratings should be made—for example, hourly, daily, or weekly. This important decision should consider (1) the frequency of the target behavior as indicated in the FBA, (2) the age of the student, and (3) natural breaks in the student's schedule.

If a problem behavior occurs frequently, ratings of the child's behavior should occur frequently as well. Children with high-rate behaviors have a better chance of succeeding when short periods between evaluative ratings are scheduled. Achieving success during one rating period may increase the child's motivation to succeed in subsequent rating periods. Rating periods that are too long will increase the likelihood that the child will fail within each rating interval, resulting in low motivation to behave appropriately in the subsequent rating period.

Student Name: _____   Teacher Signature: _____

Date: _____   Resource Rm Teacher Signature: _____

Behavior Goals:

1. Complete work accurately and completely
2. Request assistance when needed

SCHEDULE

Attendance & Sharing	YES	NO
Math	YES	NO
Music/Art	YES	NO
Social Studies	YES	NO
Unstructured Study Period	YES	NO
Recess	YES	NO
Reading	YES	NO
Lunch	YES	NO
Spelling	YES	NO
Language Arts	YES	NO
Recess	YES	NO
Science	YES	NO

Goal: /12   Total: /12

Reward: _____ (Earn a Coupon)

Comments: _____
_____
_____
_____
_____

FIGURE 5.2. Sample individual behavior rating scale. Copyright 2003 by Deanne A. Crone and Robert H. Horner. From *Building Behavior Support Systems in Schools: Functional Behavioral Assessment* by Deanne A. Crone and Robert H. Horner. Permission to photocopy this page is granted to purchasers of this book for personal use only (see copyright page for details).

Younger children require more frequent feedback than older children. Optimally, rating scales for young children should be designed to provide feedback several times within a class period (e.g., four times during a 20-minute reading lesson). Rating periods for older children can be longer (e.g., after each class period for a middle school student).

Rating periods can often fit into natural breaks in the student's schedule. For an elementary school student, each rating period could correspond to a new task—for example, circle time, language arts, and recess. For a middle school student, each rating period could correspond to the break between classes or between blocks of classes.

Once the data have been collected over a specified period of time, it should be graphed to illustrate the student's progress. Two weeks (the recommended period of time between the design of the BSP and the first follow-up meeting) is a reasonable amount of time to collect enough data to make data-based decisions about the BSP. A graph of Tom's evaluation data is illustrated in Figure 5.3.

A member of the team should share the student's graph with the student. A visual depiction of the student's behavior may mean more to the student than other means of providing feedback.

Often, the team will want to keep a record of the behavior summary sheet while providing a daily report to the student's parents. This potential paperwork problem can be resolved by using rating forms printed on duplicate or triplicate paper.

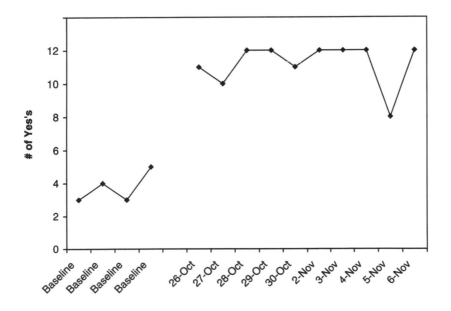

FIGURE 5.3. Graphical summary of Tom's evaluation data.

Observation

Observation is another commonly used method of evaluation. Observations are typically conducted by a member of the team who has skills in behavioral assessment. The observer notes occurrences of on-task behavior, off-task behavior, problem behaviors (as defined by the FBA), and expected behaviors (as defined by the evaluation plan; see Appendix B, Step 8: Evaluate Plan). The observation should be conducted during the routine(s) that is (are) targeted in the evaluation plan. The length of the observation is dictated by the length of the routine. The team may want to assess if a new skill has generalized to reduce problem behavior in a nonintervention routine. If so, they must collect evaluation data in nonintervention settings as well. A sample observation coding sheet was illustrated in Chapter 3 (see Figure 3.11). Figure 5.4 provides a graphic summary of observation evaluation data for the first 2 weeks after Vera's BSP was implemented.

Documenting the Evaluation Plan

The F-BSP Protocol includes a page to document the evaluation plan (see Appendix B, Step 8). Figures 5.5, 5.6, and 5.7 illustrate the evaluation plans for Vera, Ronald, and Tom. There are three key components to designing the evaluation plan: (1) deciding on the long-term and short-term behavioral goals, (2) de-

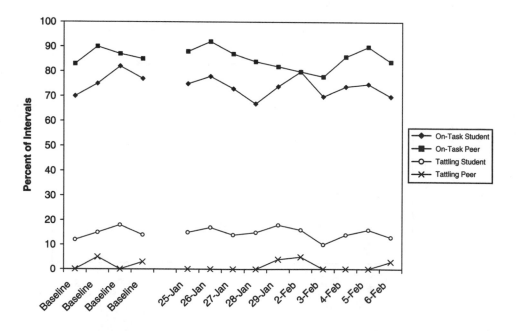

FIGURE 5.4. Summary of observation evaluation data for Vera.

Step 8: Evaluate Plan

Behavioral Goal (use specific, observable, measurable descriptions of goal)

What is the short-term behavioral goal?
For 95% or more of intervals observed, Vera will request help from teacher to solve peer conflict without engaging in "tattling," in other words, pushing, whining, or crying about other students.

<u>2/6/99</u>   Expected date

What is the long-term behavioral goal?
Share materials appropriately and work cooperatively (without tattling) with classmates for 100% of intervals

<u>3/6/99</u>   Expected date

Evaluation Procedures

Data to Be Collected	Procedures for Data Collection	Person Responsible	Timeline
Time on-task (includes working cooperatively) Time tattling Peer comparison for on-task and tattling	School psychologist does brief, daily observation during Circle Time and records graphically. Share graph with team at follow-up meeting.	School psychologist	Begin 1/25/99 until 2/6/99

Plan review date: <u>2/6/99</u>

We agree to the conditions of this plan:

Student	(date)	Parent or guardian	(date)
Teacher	(date)	Teacher	(date)
Action Team member	(date)	Action Team member	(date)

FIGURE 5.5. Evaluation plan for Vera.

Step 8: Evaluate Plan

Behavioral Goal (use specific, observable, measurable descriptions of goal)

What is the short-term behavioral goal?
For at least 10 out of 12 class periods, Tom will learn to request intermittent attention/assistance from teacher or competent peer (when needed) rather than have a tantrum

<u>11/8/99</u>   Expected date

What is the long-term behavioral goal?
For at least 10 out of 12 class periods, Tom will complete work on his own, without disruption

<u>12/15/99</u>   Expected date

Evaluation Procedures

Data to Be Collected	Procedures for Data Collection	Person Responsible	Timeline
Daily report on whether or not he met his two behavior card goals during each class period	Daily behavior report card. Make sure all staff (e.g., homeroom teacher, music teacher, etc.) understand purpose and use card consistently. Teacher responsible for filling out card on daily basis. Report data to team graphically.	School psychologist initiates and monitors	Begin immediately, 10/21/99; continue at least until review date, 11/8/99

Plan review date: <u>11/8/99</u>

We agree to the conditions of this plan:

_____		_____	
Student	(date)	Parent or guardian	(date)
_____		_____	
Teacher	(date)	Teacher	(date)
_____		_____	
Action Team member	(date)	Action Team member	(date)

FIGURE 5.6. Evaluation plan for Tom.

Step 8: Evaluate Plan

Behavioral Goal (use specific, observable, measurable descriptions of goal)

What is the short-term behavioral goal?
For 95% or more of class periods, Ronald will avoid aggressive behavior toward peers by requesting a break from group activity or requesting to work with different peers.

_2/28/99_ Expected date

What is the long-term behavioral goal?
For at least 80% of class periods, Ronald will work cooperatively and productively during structured group activity.

_6/6/99_ Expected date

Evaluation Procedures

Data to Be Collected	Procedures for Data Collection	Person Responsible	Timeline
Daily report on whether or not he met his behavior card goals during each class period with comments about requests for breaks	Daily behavior report card. Make sure all staff (e.g., homeroom teacher, music teacher, etc.) understand purpose and use card consistently. Teacher responsible for filling out card on daily basis. Report data to team graphically.	School psychologist initiates and monitors the card	Begin immediately, 2/11/99; continue at least until review date 2/28/99

Plan review date: _2/28/99_

We agree to the conditions of this plan:

Student	(date)	Parent or guardian	(date)
Teacher	(date)	Teacher	(date)
Action Team member	(date)	Action Team member	(date)

FIGURE 5.7. Evaluation plan for Ronald.

ciding how to measure if the goals have been met, and (3) documenting when the team will reconvene to examine the evaluation data and make decisions regarding whether or not to monitor, modify, or discontinue the BSP.

The long-term and short-term goals have been previously suggested by the Competing Behavior Pathway form. The long-term goal can be identified by operationally defining the "desired behavior." Likewise, the short-term goal can be derived from the "alternative behavior." These goals can be transferred to the evaluation plan page. It is important to be specific about the criterion level for reaching the goal. For example, rather than stating something like, *"Carlos will increase his work completion rate,"* the goal may be listed as *"Carlos will complete at least 50% of each assignment before the end of each class period."* Measurement of the behavior can be accomplished using any of the methods described in the previous section. A follow-up meeting to assess the impact of the behavioral strategies on the short-term and long-term behavioral goals should be scheduled to occur within 2–3 weeks.

The evaluation plan page also includes a space for the signatures of the student, parent, teacher, and action team members. By signing at the end of the F-BSP Protocol, all of the participating members indicate that they (1) understand the assessment information provided, (2) understand and agree to their responsibilities in implementing the BSP, and (3) understand and agree to the evaluation plan. Requesting these individuals to sign the F-BSP Protocol provides a means for increasing communication and collaboration among the key players involved in providing behavioral support to the identified student.

Assessing Feasibility and Fidelity of Behavior Support Plan Implementation

Poor or inconsistent implementation is a common cause of BSP failure. Evaluation data can help the team determine if the failure of a BSP is due to a failure to appropriately implement it. The simplest evaluation strategy is to ask each member of the team if he or she completed his or her role in the student's BSP. One of the strategies listed on Ronald's BSP was that the school psychologist would teach Ronald to ask for a break. The school psychologist can quickly confirm if this strategy was or was not implemented.

A quick check on implementation fidelity can be achieved by requesting each team member to briefly describe his or her role. A team member who cannot describe what he or she was expected to do has obviously not implemented his or her portion of the BSP. This situation indicates a larger, communication problem among members of the team, one that can be remedied by careful attention to collaboration, documentation, and distribution of the BSP. We recommend that on the first few days of BSP implementation, the team leader check in with each involved staff member to determine if that person has carried out his or her part of the plan. These brief check-ins are a simple way to increase accountability for BSP implementation, while also serving to detect any support needs that a staff member may experience in the initial implementation stages.

Individualized behavior rating scales can easily be used as a check on fidelity of implementation. If completed rating scales demonstrate consistent completion over a continuous period of time, the Action Team can conclude that the intervention was implemented as planned. Conversely, if the rating scales are blank, missing data, or appear to have been completed in one sitting during a "catch-up moment," the team can conclude that the intervention was not implemented as planned.

Direct observation is a time-consuming yet informative strategy to monitor implementation fidelity. Often, the BSP requires the teacher to change his or her typical responses to the target student. The teacher may be expected to ignore inappropriate behavior or to provide reinforcements for appropriate behavior. The teacher can invite a member of the team to observe his or her classroom to determine if the BSP is being implemented as planned. The observer can also act as a consultant to the teacher, providing support and suggestions for improving implementation fidelity.

Some BSP strategies will be very simple to observe. For example, Ronald's BSP indicated that he should be separated from certain peers during group projects. The observer could visit Ronald's class during a group activity and simply note if the change in physical arrangement had been completed.

The evaluation may show that significant portions of the BSP were not implemented as planned. The Behavior Support Team must determine if implementation was hampered by issues of contextual fit and subsequently work to resolve any existing problems.

Assessing Parent, Teacher, and Student Satisfaction

Consumer feedback is an important element of program development and maintenance. Consumer feedback can identify dissatisfaction with elements of the FBA-BSP process that could affect willingness to contribute and participate. Consumers can also provide perceptive suggestions for improving function-based behavior support. Students, parents, teachers, and members of the Behavior Support Team can be regularly surveyed to determine their satisfaction with, and suggestions for, the FBA-BSP process. These surveys can be used to improve services for the identified child or to improve the overall process. Sample consumer satisfaction surveys are included in Chapter 7 (see Figures 7.7, 7.8, and 7.9).

DATA-BASED DECISIONS

The Behavior Support Team should use the evaluation data to make decisions about four questions:

1. Were the goals of the behavior support plan achieved?
2. Was the intervention implemented as planned?
3. Is more assessment needed?
4. In what ways should the intervention be modified?

In the first meeting following implementation of the BSP, the team must evaluate whether the goals of the BSP were achieved. One member of the team should summarize the evaluation data in a graph and distribute copies to each member of the core team. The criterion for determining if the goals were achieved is specified by "short-term goal" and "long-term goal" in the evaluation plan. This criterion level can be indicated by the graphical summary of the evaluation data (see Figure 5.8 for an example). If the data are collected and used properly, it should be rather simple to decide if the goals of the BSP were achieved. Examine Figures 5.8 and 5.9. It is clear that the strategies in the BSP were effective in increasing Tom's appropriate behavior (Figure 5.8). In contrast, it appears that initial implementation of Ronald's BSP was unsuccessful; his behavior remained at levels far below the criterion level (Figure 5.9).

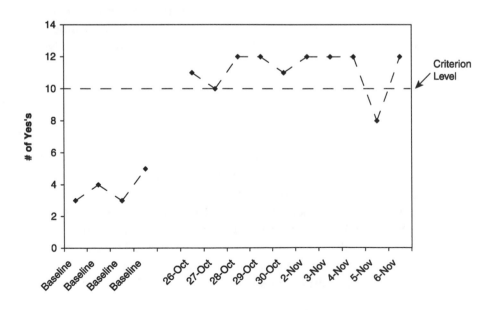

FIGURE 5.8. Evaluation data for Tom with criterion level.

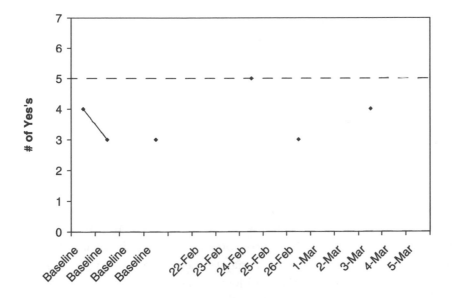

FIGURE 5.9. Summary of evaluation data for Ronald—Behavior Rating Scale.

If the goals of the BSP were not achieved, the team should assess the problem and proceed accordingly. First the team should assess whether the BSP was implemented as planned. This question is answered by examining the evaluation of implementation data. Ronald's behavior rating scale contains missing data points for seven of the 14 possible rating periods. Clearly, this strategy was not implemented with sufficient frequency or consistency. If, based on the functional behavioral assessment data, the team believes that this strategy should be an effective response to Ronald's problem behavior, the strategy should be reimplemented over the subsequent 2-week period. Prior to reimplementation, the team should examine if issues of contextual fit hinder the full implementation of the strategy and should modify the plan to meet the contextual fit needs.

The team can also evaluate the fidelity of implementation by examining observational data. Figure 5.10 presents the summary of observation data for implementation of Vera's BSP. The strategies observed are ignoring tattling behavior and praising appropriate behavior. During the interval observed, Vera's teacher ignored her tattling behavior for 90% of the behavioral events. She praised Vera for working appropriately and sharing materials for 100% of the observation intervals. From this data, it is clear that Vera's teacher implemented the BSP as planned.

Despite its fidelity of implementation, Vera's BSP did not result in reduction of tattling (refer to Figure 5.4). At this point, the team must decide if further assessment is necessary. The BSP may be built upon an erroneous hypothesis statement. For example, the team concluded that Vera tattled on fellow class-

Teacher Behavior	% of intervals	Student behavior	% of intervals
Ignore tattling behavior	90	Tattling—baseline	12
Praise appropriate sharing	100	Tattling—Day 6 intervention	15

FIGURE 5.10. Summary of implementation observation data.

mates to obtain attention from her teacher. The BSP was designed so that Vera could earn teacher attention by engaging in appropriate play with her peers. If, however, Vera tattles in order to escape her peers, the BSP intervention will simply increase her anxiety and discomfort without providing the necessary reinforcement. In such a case, the team should reconsider the function of Vera's tattling behavior (further assessment may be necessary) and redesign the BSP to match the true function of the problem behavior.

How does the team decide if additional assessment is necessary? If the BSP was implemented carefully and consistently, but progress toward the goals was not achieved, additional assessment should be considered. If failure to achieve progress toward the goals was based on a simple FBA (i.e., teacher interview only), additional assessment will be essential. Additional assessment should emphasize (1) interviewing the student to identify personally meaningful punishers and reinforcers, and (2) increasing confidence in the hypothesis statement.

MAINTENANCE PLAN

After a student has successfully achieved his or her behavioral goals, the Behavior Support Team should design a maintenance plan to ensure continued support and success for the student and his or her teacher. Students are vulnerable to losing behavioral gains as they transition from one grade level to the next. Without continued support from the new teacher, the student may quickly revert to the more familiar, baseline levels of problem behavior. To create the maintenance plan, the team should redesign the BSP for efficiency. They may choose to remove, modify, continue, or update different aspects of the BSP. The primary goal of the maintenance plan is continued success for the child while reducing the required amount of staff time and resources. The maintenance plan should be documented and distributed to each member of the team.

PART THREE

Using Functional Behavioral Assessment within School Systems: Questions and Considerations

CHAPTER 6

Who Will Be Involved in the Behavior Support Team and What Is Needed from Each Person?

INTRODUCTION

A sustainable system of individual behavior support should be built on a team-based foundation (Todd, Horner, Sugai, & Colvin, 1999). Many schools rely on one individual, such as the school psychologist, to take on the role of the behavior support specialist. This person is often an itinerant employee, based in multiple buildings during one school year, who may also switch buildings from year to year. This arrangement makes it challenging for the individual's ability to build relationships with staff and students, to understand the daily challenges and successes experienced by the school, or to build an enduring system of individual behavior support. Other schools may have an in-building behavior specialist. However, the loss of this one person to a new job, illness, or other obligation could result in the loss of the school's entire system of individual behavior support.

A team-based approach to behavior support should be established so that it can support a changing membership. Given the dynamic nature of many schools, it may be difficult to predict staff responsibilities and team participation from year to year. Even so, individuals who serve on the core individual Behavior Support Team should commit to serving on the team for at least 1 to 3 academic years. Each school should concentrate on developing within-building capacity to implement function-based behavior support so that the school can become resilient to fluctuations in team membership.

Behavior Support Teams are also dynamic in that the individuals involved in each referral will change from student to student. For example, the parents and the teacher of the referred student should be involved in the assessment and intervention process. This set of individuals will change for each new referral. The team must be structured to handle rotating parent and teacher involvement.

In this chapter we outline the structure, membership, roles, and responsibilities of the Behavior Support Team. In the remaining chapters, we outline models for building internal capacity for function-based behavior support within the school.

BEHAVIOR SUPPORT TEAM STRUCTURE

Each Behavior Support Team is unique. Teams will vary from school to school in terms of size, membership, structure, fluency, student population, and theoretical perspective. Despite these differences, all teams should share certain critical features. Todd et al. (1999) outline these features: "Teams that support students with chronic problem behaviors need to (a) possess specialized behavioral skills within their membership, (b) allow and encourage contributions from all their members, (c) have predictable and efficient procedures for doing business and solving problems, (d) have regular opportunities to access building staff, families and community agencies to communicate and solicit information" (p. 74). A team that possesses these defining features should be able to meet the following primary objectives: "(a) manage teacher requests for assistance, (b) ensure that teachers and students receive support in a timely and meaningful manner, (c) provide a general forum for discussions and possible solutions for individual student behavioral concerns, and (d) organize a collaborative effort to support the teacher" (Todd et al., 1999, p. 74).

We advocate a two-tiered model for Behavior Support Teams. The first tier is comprised of the core team members. The second tier consists of separate Action Teams for each referred student. The membership at each level is illustrated in Figure 6.1.

The core team will consist of a school administrator, an individual with behavioral expertise, and a representative sample of the school staff. The Action Team will consist of one or two members from the core team, the student's parents, the student's teacher(s) and/or the staff member who made the initial request for assistance, and any other significant persons in the student's life who wish to participate (e.g., counselor, social worker, probation officer). (In the case of referrals that require only a simple FBA, the Action Team will often be limited to the referring teacher and an individual with behavioral expertise.) At least one person on each Action Team should have expertise in FBA and individual behavior support. In the early stages of implementing FBA-BSP, there may be

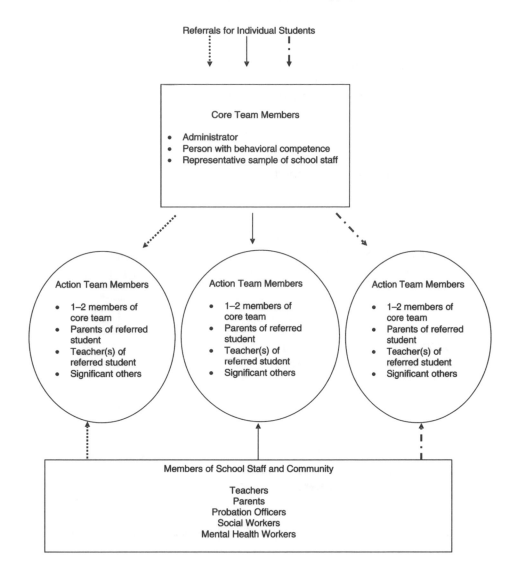

FIGURE 6.1. Diagram of the two-level team approach to function-based individual behavior support.

only one individual within a school who has this behavioral expertise. Until additional expertise is built into the within-building capacity of the school, this individual should serve on every Action Team.

The core team and the individual Action Team work together to respond to each referral. Figure 6.2 illustrates this process. The core team is responsible for receiving and managing referrals, forming and supporting Action Teams, and contributing (as needed) to the design, evaluation, and modification of BSPs. The Action Team acts as a subgroup of the core team. The Action Team collects

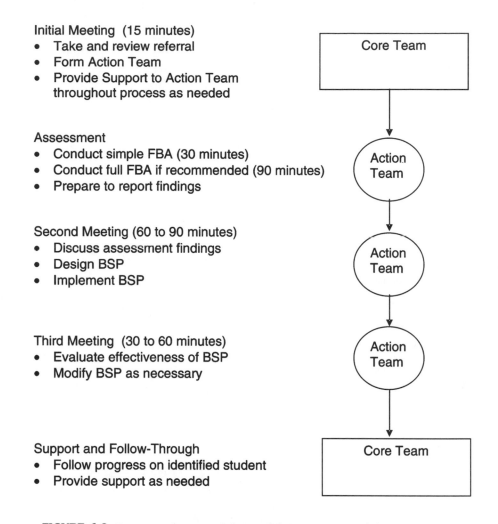

Initial Meeting (15 minutes)
- Take and review referral
- Form Action Team
- Provide Support to Action Team throughout process as needed

Assessment
- Conduct simple FBA (30 minutes)
- Conduct full FBA if recommended (90 minutes)
- Prepare to report findings

Second Meeting (60 to 90 minutes)
- Discuss assessment findings
- Design BSP
- Implement BSP

Third Meeting (30 to 60 minutes)
- Evaluate effectiveness of BSP
- Modify BSP as necessary

Support and Follow-Through
- Follow progress on identified student
- Provide support as needed

FIGURE 6.2. Process and responsibilities of the core team and the action teams.

the FBA data, leads the design and implementation of the BSP, provides support to the student and teacher before and during the implementation of the BSP, collects evaluation data on the effectiveness of the BSP on the student's behavior, and provides feedback on contextual limitations that impact the implementation of the BSP.

Membership on the core team lasts for at least 1 academic school year and often for 2 or more academic years. If core team members commit to participating for 2 or more years, the individual behavior support system should become more stable since the team will have more time and flexibility to build within-building capacity for function-based behavior support.

Membership on an individual Action Team lasts until the team is satisfied that the goals of the BSP have been achieved. Members of the Action Teams must be apprised of the expected time commitment necessary to design, implement, and evaluate an individual BSP. Although time commitments will vary depending on the needs of the student, on average the Action Team should expect the following: (1) reviewing referral and planning assessment (15-minute meeting); (2) collecting assessment data (about 30 minutes for a simple FBA and 90–120 minutes for a full FBA); (3) designing a function-based BSP (60–90-minute meeting); (4) follow-up of evaluation (30–60-minute meeting); and (5) continued meeting and support (as necessary). Action Team members must agree to this time commitment while remaining flexible enough to handle unpredictable delays or extensions.

Teachers (or other staff) who request assistance with an individual student should understand that they will be expected to become part of the Action Team for that student. Without their input and assistance, the team will not be able to gain a clear understanding of the problem, nor will they be able to implement effective solutions to the problem. In most cases, the referring teacher will be responsible for implementing some of the intervention strategies generated by the team.

Initially, in order to build expertise and fluency in function-based behavior support, all of the core team members may choose to participate on each Action Team. That is, after one or two individuals have collected assessment information, the entire core team may decide to meet with the referring teacher and/or parent to summarize the assessment information and to develop and evaluate the BSP.

BEHAVIOR SUPPORT TEAM MEMBERSHIP

Every core Behavior Support Team should incorporate a certain mix of individuals. This critical mix should include a school principal, a person with strong skills and experiences in behavioral assessment and intervention, and a representative sample of the school's personnel. The actual size of the team will vary from school to school. A typical team size may be 4 to 6 individuals. We suggest limiting the maximum size of the group to eight. Beyond eight individuals, it becomes quite cumbersome to move forward with decision making and planning.

School Principal

The principal must be an active participant on the core team. There are multiple reasons for involving an administrator on the Behavior Support Team:

1. *Courtesy*. Effective principals need to know what is going on in their schools. Serious problem behaviors of individual students are an especially sensitive issue in which the principal must be involved.

2. *Valuable input*. The administrator may have unique information to contribute to the FBA-BSP process. The administrator may have had more contact than other staff with the student's family and may be aware of important setting events for problem behaviors.

3. *Spending authority*. Administrators have spending authority over any flexible monies in the school budget. One of the critical elements in building internal capacity for individual behavior support is to allocate approximately 10 hours of employment time per 200 students to a team coordinator. If the administrator is an integral part of the Behavior Support team, she or he is much more apt to agree that this is a wise use of the school's flex money.

4. *Administrative influence*. Within a school, administrators have the power to drive change or to impede it. Administrators have the authority to approve or refuse teacher and staff requests. To illustrate, the core team may develop a BSP that requires one teacher to assist another teacher during initial implementation. The principal must decide if the first teacher can leave her own classroom to assist in the other classroom. The principal is also responsible for finding a temporary substitute for that teacher. It is much more efficient to develop the BSP with the principal's input and approval than to revise and modify a BSP after an administrative veto.

Individual with Competence in Behavioral Assessment and Intervention

There must be a person with expertise in applied behavioral analysis to guide decision making, assessment, and intervention. This person can be an outside-contracted behavioral consultant, the school psychologist, or an in-building person with training, experience, and competence. This person must have a firm knowledge of behavioral theory and its application, FBA, and behavioral intervention. It is important to avoid relying *solely* on the expertise of an outside-contracted behavioral consultant. Initially, schools may have to rely on outside expertise, but a plan should be put in place to build internal behavioral capacity within the school. In Chapter 8, we will discuss a model for building internal behavioral capacity.

Representative Sample of School Staff

The core team needs to include a representative sample of the school staff. A representative sample would include teachers of different grade levels, general and special educators, and nonteaching staff (e.g., school nurse, lunchroom monitor, etc.). A representative sample of middle or high school teachers would also cut across subject matter fields or departments. Paraprofessionals (e.g., educational assistants) that play an important role in school settings where problem behaviors often occur should also be represented on the team. For example, a recess monitor or cafeteria monitor can contribute invaluable information about the predictors and consequences of problem behaviors in these settings. Educational assistants may also have more flexible time than a classroom teacher. This flexible time can allow them to conduct observations or collect other assessment information for the FBA-BSP. Whereas the technical person is the expert in applied behavioral theory, these other team members are experts in understanding the strengths, weaknesses, and contextual limitations of their own school environment.

Parent

Some Behavior Support Teams may choose to include a parent as a permanent member of the core team. Often, a parent can offer a new and discerning perspective. Inclusion of a parent on the team reduces the tendency to blame families for problem behaviors and maintains the team's focus on altering problematic environmental routines within the school.

BEHAVIOR SUPPORT TEAM ROLES AND RESPONSIBILITIES

The members of the core Behavior Support Team will fill both management and performance roles.

Management Roles

Each Behavior Support Team will need a coordinator/referral liaison. The person who serves these functions should remain constant throughout the school year. Utilizing more than one initial-contact person may be confusing to school staff and result in underutilization of the individual behavior support system. In addition, division of responsibility for initial referrals could lead to disorganization, decreased accountability, and reduced efficiency in responding to teachers' requests for assistance. *The level of credibility of and teacher confidence in the core Behavior Support Team will sustain or ruin this system of individual behavioral support. Thus, choosing a conscientious, responsible member of the team to act as the referral liaison for the entire team is of critical importance.*

The role of coordinator/referral liaison can be filled by any member of the core team. This person should be organized, should be responsible, and should possess strong leadership and communication skills. Previous experience managing or leading a school-based team will facilitate the individual's ability to fulfill the role of coordinator, but is not necessary. The role of coordinator is not easy, nor is it always rewarding. Coordinators are typically most successful when they are intrinsically interested in individual behavioral support and are strongly committed to the success of the team. Finally, coordinators must be supported by the rest of the team members. A coordinator who has many negative relationships with other school staff will impair rather than expedite the success of the team.

The coordinator/referral liaison's role is to facilitate the FBA-BSP process. The responsibilities of this role may change as the team strengthens and builds their skills in FBA-BSP. In the initial stages of building the individual behavior support team, all of the team members may participate on each Action Team. In this case, the coordinator will need to take on a strong leadership role. The coordinator will generate an agenda for each team meeting. To increase the team's overall preparedness, the coordinator should distribute the agenda at least 1 day prior to the meeting. The coordinator will lead the meetings, and try to keep them focused and efficient. The Behavior Support Team will generate a task list for each referral (e.g., invite parent to next meeting, conduct FBA interview with teacher, etc.). The coordinator will assure that someone is responsible for the completion of each task. It is not the coordinator's role to assign tasks to members of the team. Rather, the coordinator should foster a spirit of collaboration and volunteerism among team members. If certain tasks are left unclaimed, the coordinator may ask for assistance from individual team members. The coordinator should resist the temptation to take all remaining tasks upon him- or herself. This would only create an imbalance in team involvement, as well as cause undue stress and overload to the coordinator. The coordinator should distribute a list of responsibilities to each team member. The list should identify each task, the person responsible for each task, and the expected deadline for completion of each task. This list should highlight the date of the next follow-up meeting for the referred student.

The team will also need an individual to take notes at each meeting. This responsibility can be shifted from meeting to meeting. The note taker should be sure to record any tasks that arise, deadlines, dates, and decisions made. The note taker will provide this information to the coordinator, who will then organize and distribute it.

As each team member begins to feel more comfortable in conducting FBAs and developing BSPs, the core team may move to the Action Team model described earlier. In the Action Team model, only one or two members from the core behavior support team are involved in each student referral. Once the school moves to the Action Team model, the coordinator of the core team will play a smaller role. This is because the core team members serving on each Action Team will take on the leadership responsibilities for that Action Team that were previously filled by the coordinator. The coordinator of the core team will continue to (1) receive the referrals, (2) distribute the referral to one or two core team members who will form an Action Team for that student, (3) follow up on the progress of the Action Team, and (4) maintain a copy of the assessment data and records generated by the Action Team.

Performance Roles

Performance roles are dictated by the tasks that need to be completed. These roles include: (1) conducting FBA interviews and observations, (2) reviewing academic records and work samples, (3) reporting FBA data to the larger group, (4) generating testable hypotheses, and (5) designing, implementing, evaluating, and modifying BSPs. The individuals who complete these tasks can rotate from referral to referral. Once each team member has developed skill in conducting FBA assessment and intervention, he or she will be able to lead an individual Action Team. These individuals will conduct the interviews and observations for a specific referral. Ideally, every member of the core team should be skilled in interviewing, observing, reporting, designing, evaluating, and monitoring. Achieving this goal will take time, commitment, and training. Until team members are adequately skilled, a behavior consultant or the school psychologist may complete all of the FBAs while the team contributes to the design and implementation of the BSP. Refer to Chapters 7 and 8 for information on how to build a school-based team with FBA-BSP skills.

CHAPTER 7

How Do You Get the Behavior Support Team to Work Together as a Team?

INTRODUCTION

Todd et al. (1999) assert that a *team-based* approach is critical to implementing a sustainable, efficient system of individual behavior support within schools: "Unlike a system that is led by a single individual, a team-based approach can be sustained when staff members join and leave a staff, difficult decisions must be made, and major effort must be directed toward implementation of a project" (p. 73). A function-based approach to individual behavior support will be a new approach to behavior management for most schools and most behavior support teams. It will take time, effort, and patience to become effective and efficient as a team. A strong organizational structure and process will lay the foundation for building an effective, efficient team, and will maintain the team as it develops and grows. Critical features of an effective team with strong organizational structure include: (1) efficient use of time, (2) high profile within the school, (3) consistent participation, (4) efficient system of documentation, (5) clear organizing procedure that delineates roles and responsibilities, (6) system of accountability for responsibilities, and (7) a clearly defined system for making data-based decisions. These features will be discussed in detail in the present chapter.

ORGANIZING STRUCTURE

A basic organizing structure will go a long way in getting a team to work to-gether. An organizing structure should (1) keep the team focused on their objec-tives, (2) keep the team moving forward toward real (observable and measur-able) outcomes, and (3) give the team a record of where they began and how much progress has been made.

Everyone has been in a meeting that seemed to drag on without providing any useful information or resulting in any decisions. After one or two meetings like this, team members begin to avoid attending meetings or participating on that committee. One of the most serious obstacles to implementation of individ-ual behavior support is limited staff time. Team members cannot afford to waste time in inefficient disorganized meetings.

How do you run an efficient meeting? Begin with an agenda. Without an or-ganizing focus, groups tend to stray off the topic, especially when the topic is se-rious problem behaviors. The best way to regain momentum is to focus the group on the agenda and the objectives that must be achieved within the allot-ted time. The content of each agenda will vary depending on what stage the team is at in responding to a referral. As discussed in Chapter 6, the team will meet at least three times in responding to a referral: (1) after the initial referral, (2) after the Action Team has collected functional assessment data, and (3) after the behavior support plan has been implemented for at least 2 weeks. Figures 7.1, 7.2, and 7.3 illustrate sample agendas for each of these meetings. On many occasions, the Behavior Support Team may be working on more than one refer-ral at a time, and may well be at different stages with each referral. As time per-mits, the agendas illustrated in Figures 7.1, 7.2, and 7.3 can be combined into one meeting for more than one student, to fit the needs of the Behavior Support Team.

The agenda should include time limits for each agenda item. Placing time limits on the discussion of each item helps the team prioritize and complete the objectives of the meeting. It is too easy to persist on one point and not complete the entire agenda. Items that are not addressed in one meeting will have to be added to the agenda of the next meeting. School-based teams do not have the luxury of waiting an additional week or two to respond to a teacher's request for assistance. Serious problem behaviors pose possible safety or health issues for the school. Delaying assistance because the team persisted on one agenda item will be unacceptable to the teacher in need.

The length of the team meeting will vary depending on whether it is a plan-ning meeting, a BSP design meeting, or a follow-up meeting. The length of the meeting will also depend on how skilled the team is in completing each stage of function-based behavior support. Throughout the year, as teams have more op-

BEHAVIOR SUPPORT TEAM AGENDA

Date: _____

Student: _____ (Initials only)

I. Introductions (introduce selves to parents or other new members and summarize purpose of meeting)—5 minutes

II. Review Request for Assistance—5 minutes

III. Determine level of functional assessment to begin with (simple or full)—2 minutes

IV. Form Action Team—1 minute

V. Assign responsibilities and deadlines for completing FBA—2 minutes

FIGURE 7.1. Sample agenda—Initial meeting. From *Building Positive Behavior Support Systems in Schools: Functional Behavioral Assessment* by Deanne A. Crone and Robert H. Horner. Copyright 2003 by The Guilford Press. Permission to photocopy this figure is granted to purchasers of this book for personal use only (see copyright page for details).

ACTION TEAM AGENDA

Date: _____

Student: _____ (Initials only)

I. Action Team reports data from simple FBA or full FBA—15 minutes

II. Develop testable hypothesis—10 minutes

III. Determine if further FBA or functional analysis is required—2 minutes

IV. If further assessment is not required, design BSP—20 minutes

V. Design plan for implementation of BSP—5–10 minutes

VI. Determine method of data collection for evaluation of behavior support plan—5 to 10 minutes

VII. Schedule follow-up meeting—1 minute

FIGURE 7.2. Sample agenda—Second meeting. *Note*: This is a great deal of work to complete in 1 hour. If the team is available for longer, we suggest extending this meeting to 90 minutes and expanding the amount of time allowed for each activity accordingly. From *Building Positive Behavior Support Systems in Schools: Functional Behavioral Assessment* by Deanne A. Crone and Robert H. Horner. Copyright 2003 by The Guilford Press. Permission to photocopy this figure is granted to purchasers of this book for personal use only (see copyright page for details).

BEHAVIOR SUPPORT TEAM AGENDA

Date: _____

Student: _____ (Initials only)

I. Action team reports on implementation and impact of BSP—5–10 minutes

II. Determine if BSP goals were achieved—2 minutes

III. Determine if BSP modification is necessary—2 minutes

IV. Modify BSP and evaluation plan as necessary—10–15 minutes

V. Schedule follow-up plan as necessary—1 minute

FIGURE 7.3. Sample agenda—Third Meeting. *Note*: This is a great deal of work to complete in 30 minutes. If the team is available for longer, we suggest extending this meeting to 60 minutes and expanding the amount of time allowed for each activity accordingly. From *Building Positive Behavior Support Systems in Schools: Functional Behavioral Assessment* by Deanne A. Crone and Robert H. Horner. Copyright 2003 by The Guilford Press. Permission to photocopy this figure is granted to purchasers of this book for personal use only (see copyright page for details).

portunities to practice, they will become more fluent in the process. We suggest that the team coordinator allocate 15 minutes to the planning meeting, at least 1 hour to the assessment summary and BSP design meeting, and at least 30 minutes for the follow-up/evaluation meeting. Figures 7.1, 7.2, and 7.3 include approximate time limits for discussion of each agenda item.

Using a stopwatch to keep time is an effective strategy for completing each objective on the agenda on time. At the beginning of each meeting, one person volunteers to be the timekeeper. After the coordinator introduces a new agenda item, the timekeeper reminds the group: *"We have 10 minutes to report the functional behavioral assessment data."* When there is 1 minute left to complete an item, the timekeeper tells the group to finish discussion on the first agenda item and move on to the next one. We have found that school-based teams adapt quite readily to using a stopwatch to move the agenda forward.

Full team attendance and participation should be encouraged by holding regularly scheduled meetings at the same time on the same day of the week. The frequency of meetings will be determined by the number of referrals the team receives. A bimonthly, rather than a weekly, meeting may be sufficient in a school that has a limited number of referrals. The core team will have to decide on the most convenient time for a regular meeting. Many behavior support teams prefer to meet immediately before or after school. In some school districts, the children start school an hour late, once a week. This weekly "late-start" is used by the teachers to participate in committee meetings or to prepare weekly lesson plans. It is also an opportune time to hold a behavior support team meeting.

The coordinator will generate the agenda for each team meeting. Distribution of the agenda prior to the meeting will serve as a reminder to each team member to complete his or her responsibilities and to come to the meeting prepared with all necessary materials. Many schools have established an in-house e-mail system. E-mail is a convenient, efficient means to distribute the meeting agenda to each team member. Whether the agenda is distributed via e-mail or on paper, the coordinator must be careful to maintain student confidentiality. The best way to do this is to assign an identification number to each student who is referred. An alternate choice is to use the student's initials rather than the student's full name.

A note taker should take notes at each meeting. The notes should include a brief summary of each agenda item, including any decisions that were made and any tasks or deadlines that were assigned. An example of a notes form is included in Figure 7.4. Meeting notes should be kept in a three-ring binder and stored in a confidential location that can be easily accessed by members of the team. A written record of each meeting will increase the logical flow between meetings and reduce redundant discussion and decision-making.

ORGANIZING PROCEDURE

In addition to an underlying organizational structure, the team will need an organizing procedure to follow. This procedure should delineate the team's actions from the initiation to the conclusion of each referral. The process should be efficient and responsive.

The FBA-BSP process begins when a referral is made for a student with serious problem behaviors. Typically, the initial referral is made by a teacher, but requests for assistance can be made by any staff person, parent, or the student him- or herself. The referring person completes a Request for Assistance Form. These forms should be available from the core team coordinator. It should be easy to access these forms and this person; for this reason, the coordinator should not be a parent volunteer or an itinerant employee who is in the building only once or twice a week. The Request for Assistance Form should provide (1) identifying information about the referred student; (2) information about the problem behaviors; and (3) a list of strategies that the teacher has used in the past to address the student's behavior. Directions for completing and returning the form should be clear. It should require less than 10 minutes of teacher time

Date: _____   Note Taker: _____

Present: (Fill in names of all those present)

Student: _____ (Initials only)

Agenda Item: _____
Discussion:

Decision:

Agenda Item: _____
Discussion:

Decision:

Agenda Item: _____
Discussion:

Decision:

FIGURE 7.4. Sample—Meeting Notes Form. Copyright 2003 by Deanne A. Crone and Robert H. Horner. From *Building Positive Behavior Support Systems in Schools: Functional Behavioral Assessment* by Deanne A. Crone and Robert H. Horner. Permission to photocopy this page is granted to purchasers of this book for personal use only (see copyright page for details).

to complete the Request for Assistance Form. An example Request for Assistance Form is included in Appendix A.

The teacher may require immediate, short-term assistance in addition to the long-term assistance provided by the Behavior Support Team. This is the case any time the student poses a danger to him- or herself or to others—for example, a child who engages in repetitive head banging or a child who threatens another child with a weapon. Every school should have a crisis plan in place for physically dangerous behavior. Typically, these plans involve temporarily removing the student to a "safe area." For resources on developing and implementing crisis plans, refer to the Supplementary Section at the end of Chapter 1. The crisis plan is only a temporary solution to the child's problem behavior. It is a "bandage" to be used until the team can develop and implement a long-term solution to changing the student's pattern of problem behavior.

The referring teacher or staff member should be invited to the first meeting. The core team may also want to invite the parent(s) to the planning meeting. In some cases, the core team may be discussing more than one student at a meeting. In such a case, the parent(s) should only be invited to the portion of the meeting that concerns their son or daughter. At the first meeting (the planning meeting), the core team will review the Request for Assistance. The team coordinator will request or assign one or two members from the core team to be part of the Action Team for this referral. Decisions regarding who serves on which Action Team can be based on multiple criteria:

1. Initially, there may only be one team member with expertise in FBA-BSP. Until other team members develop proficiency in FBA-BSP, this person (often the school psychologist or behavior support specialist) will have to lead every Action Team.
2. Team members may prefer to lead Action Teams for referrals from a particular grade or department. For example, a first-grade teacher may prefer to do FBA interviews with other primary grade teachers because he or she may know those teachers and those students better than the third-, fourth-, or fifth-grade students.
3. Team members may choose to rotate responsibility so that each team member participates on an equal number of Action Teams.

The core team determines which other individuals should be included in the Action Team and identifies who will invite them to participate. It is essential to include the referring teacher or staff member on the Action Team. The parents should be invited to be part of the Action Team. It is assumed that the parents can agree or disagree to participate. Sometimes, the student may be receiving additional services through a speech pathologist, social worker, or other specialist. If feasible, it is often useful to include these individuals as well. The planning meeting concludes by scheduling the next Action Team meeting (usually within a week to 10 days of the planning meeting). The note-taker puts a copy of the meeting notes in the team's three-ring binder and the meeting is adjourned. After the meeting, the team coordinator should distribute a list of responsibilities to everyone on the core team. The planning meeting should be brief, lasting 15 minutes or less.

The referring teacher, core team members, and other members of the Action Team must agree to work together as partners to develop, implement, and evaluate a BSP. We suggest formalizing this agreement by having all the members of the Action Team sign a Partnership Agreement. The purpose of the Partnership Agreement is to (1) inform Action Team members of their roles, (2) hold Action Team members accountable for their part, (3) facilitate collaboration and cooperation among members of the Action Team, and (4) ensure successful implementation and evaluation of the BSP. An example Partnership Agreement Form is included in Figure 7.5.

Before the next Action Team meeting, the core team member(s) who was (were) assigned to the Action Team will complete an FBA interview with the referring staff member. The interview should be guided by the information reported on the Request for Assistance Form. The purpose of the interview is (1) to make an immediate contact with the referring teacher, (2) to get a verbal report of the problem behavior, and (3) to obtain information on the typical setting events, predictors, and consequences of the problem behaviors.

Next, the Action Team must decide if the data collected in the simple FBA (teacher interview) is adequate or if a full FBA is necessary. This decision can be made by the team member who interviewed the referring teacher or through informal discussion with other Behavior Support Team members. A formal meeting does not need to be convened to make this decision.

As outlined in Figure 2.5, this decision is based on the following two questions:

1. Is the student at risk for suspension, expulsion or alternative school placement?
2. Are we confident that the testable hypothesis (generated from the simple FBA is correct?

If the answer to the first question is no and the answer to the second question is yes, the simple FBA is probably adequate. The Action Team should meet to develop a BSP to address the student's problem behavior. The Action Team should also determine how to implement and monitor the effectiveness of the plan. If the simple FBA is inadequate, a full FBA must be completed.

The Behavior Support Team receives referrals for students exhibiting recurring or serious problem behaviors at school. The team attempts to meet the following primary objectives: (1) manage referrals, (2) ensure that teachers and students receive support in a timely and meaningful manner, (3) provide a forum for discussions and solutions for individual student behavioral concerns, and (4) organize a collaborative effort to support the teacher and student. These objectives are met through a problem solving approach called functional behavioral assessment-based behavior support planning (FBA-BSP). The Behavior Support Team will form an Action Team to meet the needs of each referred student. The Action Team will consist of the student's teacher, parents, 1–2 members of the Behavior Support Team, and any additional persons that should be included (e.g., social worker, speech pathologist, etc.).

In order to receive support from the Behavior Support Team, teachers must agree to do the following:

1. Participate in a brief interview about the identified student
2. Provide any additional information requested by the Action Team (e.g., work samples).
3. Allow members of the Action Team to observe the student.
4. Attend Action Team meetings for the identified student.
5. Contribute to the design and implementation of a behavior support plan.
6. Collect evaluation data to document student progress after implementation of a behavior support plan.
7. Maintain the student's confidentiality.

The Behavior Support Team agrees to do the following:

1. Conduct interviews and observations in a timely and professional manner.
2. Form an Action Team to provide individualized assessment, intervention, and support for the teacher and student.
3. Design time-efficient interventions based on research-based best practices.
4. Design time-efficient methods of data collection for evaluation.
5. Report data documenting student's progress to the student, teacher, and parents.
6. Solicit teacher, student, and parent input in the assessment, intervention, and evaluation processes.
7. Modify the behavior support plan as necessary.

Action Team Member	Relation to Student	Date
Action Team Member	Relation to Student	Date
Action Team Member	Relation to Student	Date
Action Team Member	Relation to Student	Date

FIGURE 7.5. Sample Partnership Agreement Form. From *Building Positive Behavior Support Systems in Schools: Functional Behavioral Assessment* by Deanne A. Crone and Robert H. Horner. Copyright 2003 by The Guilford Press. Permission to photocopy this page is granted to purchasers of this book for personal use only (see copyright page for details).

If a full FBA must be conducted, the next step is to schedule appointments to collect further assessment data. These appointments are written down on the notes form. The full FBA is completed and the assessment person prepares to report the assessment findings to the rest of the Action Team.

The Action Team attends the second meeting (additional members of the core team can attend, but are not required to do so). The assessment person reports the full FBA data. As a group, the Action Team develops a testable hypothesis to explain why and under what circumstances the problem behavior is occurring. Once again, the team asks:

1. Are we confident that the testable hypothesis is correct
2. If we are wrong about the testable hypothesis, would the consequences be severe?

If additional information is needed, the team must ask themselves if they have the resources and expertise to conduct a functional analysis. If they do, an individual on the Action Team or an outside behavior consultant is assigned to conduct a functional analysis of behavior. If the school does not have the resources to do a functional analysis, the team may decide instead to collect additional observation or interview data to firm up their testable hypothesis. If no additional information is needed, the Action Team designs a BSP from the full FBA.

The BSP must specify individual responsibilities, timelines, and deadlines. Many times the teacher will need initial intensive support, in the beginning, to implement the BSP. This support will often come from the school psychologist, behavior support specialist, or a core behavior support team member. The Action Team also decides on a method of data collection for evaluating the effectiveness of the BSP. Before the conclusion of the second meeting, a follow-up meeting is scheduled. After the meeting, the leader of the Action Team distributes a copy of the meeting notes and the BSP to everyone on the Action Team. A copy is also placed in the core Behavior Support Team's files.

Between the BSP design meeting and the follow-up meeting, the BSP is implemented and evaluation data is collected. Before the Action Team reconvenes for the third meeting (follow-up meeting), the Action Team leader distributes the new agenda. At this meeting, the members of the Action Team report on the implementation and the evaluation of the BSP. The Action Team decides:

1. Were the goals of the behavior support plan achieved?
2. Does the behavior support plan need to be modified?

If necessary, the Action Team modifies the BSP. Once again the meeting notes (and modified BSP) are completed and distributed. If the BSP was modified, a follow-up meeting is scheduled to evaluate the effectiveness of the modified plan. If the Action Team decides that no modifications are needed, no follow-up meetings are scheduled. However, the leader of the Action Team should check in with the teacher from time to time to monitor if behavioral gains are maintained or if the teacher requires additional support.

At the end of the function-based behavior support process, the student, the teacher, and the parents can be surveyed to evaluate their level of satisfaction with the support received. Examples of Consumer Satisfaction Surveys for parents, students, and teachers, respectively, are included in Figures 7.6, 7.7, and 7.8. Feedback from these surveys should be used to improve the team's responsiveness for future referrals.

FOLLOW-UP SURVEY: PARENT FORM

1. The goals of the behavior support plan addressed my concerns about my child's behavior.

   Strongly Agree   Strongly Disagree

      1   2   3   4   5

2. The goals of the behavior support plan addressed my concerns about my child's academic progress.

   Strongly Agree   Strongly Disagree

      1   2   3   4   5

3. The suggestions made by the team were helpful.

   Strongly Agree   Strongly Disagree

      1   2   3   4   5

4. The suggestions made by the team were manageable to implement at home.

   Strongly Agree   Strongly Disagree

      1   2   3   4   5

5. I implemented the team's suggestions consistently and continuously.

   Strongly Agree   Strongly Disagree

      1   2   3   4   5

6. I have seen an improvement in my child's behavior since the behavior support plan was implemented.

   Large Improvement   No Improvement

      1   2   3   4   5

7. I have seen an improvement in my child's academic progress since the behavior support plan was implemented.

   Large Improvement   No Improvement

      1   2   3   4   5

8. I felt that my opinion and input were respected and useful to the team.

   Strongly Agree   Strongly Disagree

      1   2   3   4   5

9. Please list any other comments, concerns, or questions.

FOLLOW-UP SURVEY: STUDENT FORM

1. I was informed about the goals and procedures of the behavior support plan.

   Strongly Agree   Strongly Disagree
       1   2   3   4   5

2. I agreed that the goals of the behavior support plan were important.

   Strongly Agree   Strongly Disagree
       1   2   3   4   5

3. I agreed with the procedures that were developed for the behavior support plan.

   Strongly Agree   Strongly Disagree
       1   2   3   4   5

4. My opinions and input were requested and respected.

   Strongly Agree   Strongly Disagree
       1   2   3   4   5

5. The suggestions made by the team were consistently implemented at school.

   Strongly Agree   Strongly Disagree
       1   2   3   4   5

6. The suggestions made by the team were consistently implemented at home.

   Strongly Agree   Strongly Disagree
       1   2   3   4   5

7. I feel that my behavior has improved since the beginning of the behavior support plan.

   Large Improvement   No Improvement
       1   2   3   4   5

8. I feel that my academic skills have improved since the beginning of the behavior support plan.

   Large Improvement   No Improvement
       1   2   3   4   5

9. I would like to continue working with my teacher, parents, and the team.

   Strongly Agree   Strongly Disagree
       1   2   3   4   5

10. Please list any other comments, concerns, or questions.

FIGURE 7.7. Student Consumer Satisfaction Survey. From *Building Positive Behavior Support Systems in Schools: Functional Behavioral Assessment* by Deanne A. Crone and Robert H. Horner. Copyright 2003 by The Guilford Press. Permission to photocopy this page is granted to purchasers of this book for personal use only (see copyright page for details).

FOLLOW-UP SURVEY: TEACHER FORM

1. The goals of the behavior support plan addressed my concerns about ____'s behavior.

   Strongly Agree   Strongly Disagree
       1   2   3   4   5

2. The goals of the behavior support plan addressed my concerns about ____'s academic progress.

   Strongly Agree   Strongly Disagree
       1   2   3   4   5

3. The suggestions made by the team were helpful.

   Strongly Agree   Strongly Disagree
       1   2   3   4   5

4. The suggestions made by the team were manageable to implement in my classroom.

   Strongly Agree   Strongly Disagree
       1   2   3   4   5

5. I implemented the team's suggestions consistently and continuously.

   Strongly Agree   Strongly Disagree
       1   2   3   4   5

6. I have seen an improvement in _____'s behavior since the behavior support plan was implemented.

   Strongly Agree   Strongly Disagree
       1   2   3   4   5

7. I have seen an improvement in _____'s academic progress since the behavior support plan was implemented.

   Strongly Agree   Strongly Disagree
       1   2   3   4   5

8. Do you need any more help from the team?

9. Please list any other comments, concerns, or questions.

FIGURE 7.8. Teacher Consumer Satisfaction Survey. From *Building Positive Behavior Support Systems in Schools: Functional Behavioral Assessment* by Deanne A. Crone and Robert H. Horner. Copyright 2003 by The Guilford Press. Permission to photocopy this page is granted to purchasers of this book for personal use only (see copyright page for details).

CHAPTER 8

How Do You Generate within-Building Capacity for FBA on the Behavior Support Team?

INTRODUCTION

Each school that endeavors to meet the legislative demands of IDEA (1997) should develop a schoolwide plan to meet the following objectives: (1) provide school personnel with knowledge about the function of, assessment of, and intervention for serious behavior problems; (2) provide school personnel with strategies to conduct FBAs; (3) provide school personnel with strategies to design, implement, evaluate, and modify effective BSPs; (4) train enough individuals within a school to have the skills to complete behavioral assessment and intervention; and (5) implement a model by which efficient, effective, and relevant behavioral support can be embedded within existing school systems.

Each of these objectives emphasizes the need to generate within-building capacity for behavioral assessment and intervention. In this chapter, we discuss a strategy for promoting within-building capacity. As within-building capacity evolves, schools may choose to adopt one of several different models of leadership for their Behavior Support Team. At the end of this chapter, three models of team leadership are outlined.

The Challenge

The 1997 amendments to IDEA explicitly recommend that schools should have the capacity to use FBA in their behavior management and disciplinary actions. Unfortunately, many school personnel are unaware of this technology or lack the skills and resources to implement it. The pressure generated by the need to be in compliance with IDEA (1997) can create two serious problems: (1) haphazard, ineffective implementation of FBA-BSP; or (2) excessive spending for service contracts with behavioral consultants. The immediate challenge is to transform the current lack of skills and resources in behavioral assessment and intervention by making FBA an accessible technology that can be applied in typical school settings. Alarmingly, comprehensive training for school personnel to assume these roles is often unavailable and not competency-based.

The Goal

Simply providing the "technology" (i.e., FBA-BSP) to manage problem behaviors in schools is not enough. We also need to provide the necessary resources for its successful implementation. The schools' resources for managing problem behavior must be improved by increasing the array of individuals qualified to conduct meaningful assessments of problem behavior and to contribute to the design of effective, efficient, and relevant BSPs.

REQUIREMENTS AND COMMITMENTS

Prior to implementation, schools should be willing to commit to the following four criteria:

1. Improving behavior support systems must be established as one of the school's top three priorities and must be backed by administrative support.
2. A team should be established to assess and intervene with students who have serious behavior problems.
3. Each school should be willing to allot adequate time and resources for the team to be trained, and for the team to plan, design, and implement individual behavioral support.
4. Each school should make a commitment of at least 3 years to improving the individual behavioral support system within the school.

Without these commitments, successful efforts to train staff in behavioral assessment and intervention will be hampered.

Priorities

The function of the public school system used to be much simpler. Schools existed to provide children with an education. In the past 30 years, the "job description" of schools has expanded rapidly. Schools are now responsible for moral development, child protection, adult education, behavior management, even health care. Schools have limited resources and limited funds. It is difficult, if not impossible, for one system to effectively fill all of these roles. To be successful in one or two areas, school administrators must prioritize their goals.

Most schools can achieve an effective, efficient system of behavior support, but only if behavior support is one of the school's top priorities for at least 3 years. Weak efforts at implementing behavior support will result in frustration and wasted time. Without a serious commitment to individual behavior support, the school is better off investing its resources and efforts elsewhere. With prioritization and commitment, substantial positive changes should occur.

Commitment to individual behavior support can be demonstrated and fostered through multiple actions. First, schools can make a written commitment by including individual behavior support as a top priority in their annual school improvement plan. Administrators can support individual behavior support by encouraging and facilitating staff participation. Flexible money in the school budget can be allocated to the development and maintenance of an individual behavior support team. School staff can volunteer to serve on the team or can utilize the team by making appropriate referrals. School staff can be cooperative in the assessment process and instrumental in the intervention process. Team members and other school staff can engage in frequent discussion about how to improve the system. School staff can remain flexible and supportive as the team evolves, learns, and improves.

Resources

Adequate allocation of time and money is critical to the success of the individual behavior support team. Time and money are typically the scarcest resources in many schools. Resources must be used wisely.

Time

School psychologists and school administrators often cite "lack of time" as the biggest obstacle to implementing FBA-BSP in their schools. We believe the best way to address this limitation is through *increased efficiency* of the individual behavior support team and system. Throughout this manual, we have discussed several strategies to make the best use of limited staff time. These strategies are summarized in Table 8.1. One strategy that warrants further discussion is "making the best use of existing school-based teams."

In some cases, creating a new team may be unnecessary if an existing school-based team could be expanded or modified. Student Study Teams or

TABLE 8.1. Strategies for Making the Best Use of Time

- Implement schoolwide systems of behavior support to act as a proactive screening process for referrals.
- Determine whether each referral to the individual behavior support team is valid.
- Determine the extent of FBA that is necessary: simple FBA, full FBA, or functional analysis.
- Generate an agenda for each meeting.
- Distribute the agenda prior to each meeting to remind team members to complete tasks and to come to the meeting prepared with all necessary materials.
- Attach time limits to each agenda item.
- Use a stopwatch to enforce time limits.
- Keep notes at each meeting.
- Keep all agendas, notes, and other relevant materials in a three-ring binder in a confidential, central location.
- Meet at the same time on the same day of the week.
- Assign a within-building staff member to be the referral liaison.
- Use a wall-size calendar to remind team members of deadlines, follow-up meetings, and the like.
- Make the best use of existing school-based teams.

their equivalent (e.g., Teacher Assistance Team, Mainstream Assistance Team) have become a common feature of many schools' infrastructure. The Student Study Team typically serves a similar function to that of the individual behavior support team described in this book and typically consists of a similar cross section of school staff: general education and special education teachers from a representative portion of grade levels, the school psychologist, a counselor and/or the principal. Students who are referred to the Student Study Team may be struggling academically or behaviorally. After considering the student's needs, the Student Study Team generates, implements, and monitors an intervention plan. Unfortunately, many members of the Student Study Team are not trained in FBA or BSP design. Members of this team will need training if they are to become the core team for function-based behavior support.

Assessment and use of existing teams is recommended for at least two reasons. First, efficient use of time is a high-priority concern among school staff. Many teachers, paraprofessionals, and principals feel that they are already overcommitted. Creating a new team that serves a similar function as an existing team will be perceived (appropriately so) as an unnecessary drain on staff time and resources. Second, if two school teams serve similar purposes, but do not communicate with each other, they are likely to develop different intervention plans. Consequently, the two teams may well work at cross-purposes to each other. Teachers seeking assistance will feel caught in the middle and unsupported. The teachers' natural response will be to cease requesting assistance from either team.

We suggest increasing the schools' resources for managing problem behavior by using three strategies:

1. If a school has an existing Student Study Team, use that team to coordinate the individual behavior support system within the school. Do not create a new team.
2. Increase the school's internal capacity for behavioral expertise by providing training in function-based behavior support to members of the schools' Student Study Team.
3. Include paraprofessionals as important contributors to the team. The use of paraprofessionals in the FBA-BSP process could significantly increase the "number of hands" schools have available to conduct teacher, student, and parent interviews, and to do multiple classroom observations. Paraprofessionals could also improve the schools' capability to monitor the implementation and outcome of behavior support planning.

Financial Budget

In order to be truly effective in building a school's capacity for individual behavior support, the school or district will need to allocate financial resources to achieve this goal. The budget will vary from school to school and will depend on multiple factors, including (1) number of students, (2) number of staff, (3) magnitude of problem behaviors experienced at school, (4) current number of staff with behavioral competence, and (5) model of behavioral training implemented. At least four important pieces should be built into the budget for individual behavior support: (1) part of an individual's employment allocated to lead and coordinate the activities of the individual behavior support team, (2) money for release dollars to allow teachers and staff to attend FBA-BSP development workshops and to implement their FBA-BSP training in the school, (3) compensation for FBA-BSP development trainers, and (4) materials to support the system of individual behavior support (e.g., forms, reinforcers, curricula, etc.).

Continuum of Behavior Support Systems

A system of individual behavior support will work best in a school that has established a continuum of behavior support systems. Recall from Chapter 1 that there are at least four major behavioral systems within a school: (1) schoolwide, (2) classroom, (3) non-classroom-specific settings, and (4) individual. Students can be grouped into one of four behavioral categories: (1) students with mild or no problem behaviors, (2) students at risk for problem behaviors, (3) students with chronic patterns of problem behavior, and (4) students with dangerous problem behaviors. Valuable time and resources will be saved if the behavioral support system within a school incorporates elements for all four groups of students across all four behavioral systems. Implementing a schoolwide behavior plan such as the Effective Behavior Support

Model is an effective way to meet this ambitious goal. Additional information on the Effective Behavior Support Model can be obtained by contacting either author of this book. The basic philosophy of the Effective Behavior Support Model is described briefly below.

The majority of students (80–85%) do not need individualized behavioral support, but will respond well to simple, universal interventions (e.g., define, teach, and reward five basic rules for appropriate behavior). If the school has an effective schoolwide system in place for the majority of students, and a targeted-group-intervention system in place for the at-risk students, then only those students who truly require individualized behavioral support will be referred to the individual behavior support team. The schoolwide and targeted-group-intervention systems act as a screening process for the individual behavior support team. By increasing the validity of each referral and by reducing the overall number of referrals received, the team can be more effective and efficient. The individual behavior support team will not be able to handle all problem behaviors that are raised, especially by those students with dangerous problem behavior. For these students, the school will need to have access to additional, community services (e.g., counseling and other wraparound services).

Many schools will not have an effective continuum of behavioral support already in place. Patience, planning, and adequate allocation of resources will be essential. (Refer to the Supplementary Section of this chapter for references on schoolwide systems of behavioral support.) A behavior support team that attempts to respond to every individual behavioral issue within a school will quickly become overwhelmed, will flounder, and will fail. Therefore, in a school that does not have an established schoolwide system of behavioral support, the team will need to be very careful about deciding which referrals are valid and correspond to the group of students who require individualized support. We recommend that a school conduct a full FBA-BSP with no more than 1–5% of their student population.

A MODEL FOR GENERATING WITHIN-BUILDING CAPACITY

Expected Training Outcomes

Initially, a behavioral consultant may be the only member of the Behavior Support Team with expertise in FBA and behavior support planning. To build a team that is sustainable, the other members of the team will need to receive training that provides content and practical experience in (1) conducting FBAs, (2) designing BSPs, and (3) embedding the function-based behavior support process within the school's current structure. After training, team members should be able to demonstrate competency in several areas. *Competency* is defined as having knowledge of, and being able to demonstrate mastery of, a skill. The competencies that team members should be able to demonstrate include:

- Defining roles and responsibilities of team members.
- Defining problem behaviors in observable and measurable terms.
- Understanding setting events, antecedents, and consequences of behaviors.
- Understanding the function of a behavior.
- Developing a routine matrix.
- Interviewing students, teachers, and parents about problem behaviors.
- Observing problem behaviors in classroom and non-classroom-specific settings.
- Reporting assessment data to a team.
- Developing testable hypotheses from assessment data.
- Brainstorming intervention strategies based on the Competing Behaviors Model.
- Designing BSPs.
- Implementing, monitoring, evaluating, and modifying BSPs.

The Training Model

By providing members of the individual behavior support team with adequate training, supervision, and support, their impact on individual students will improve and their usefulness as a resource to the school will increase. Leighton et al. (1997, pp. v–vi) recommend several activities that should be applied in effective training: "1) formal orientation that sets the foundation for the individual's work; 2) training sessions that supplement and enhance knowledge and skill development, and; 3) structured, on-the-job coaching in classrooms or other learning environments."

Each school must be willing to allot adequate time and resources for the team to be trained, and for the team to plan, design, and implement FBA-BSP. For example, the administrator must be willing to release the team members from daily duties to attend training sessions.

The school or school district will need to be resourceful in locating an individual to conduct the training. If a school has already contracted for the services of a behavioral consultant, this person may be the most logical and accessible choice. The Functional Assessment Work Group at the University of Oregon has developed a set of training materials for training teams and team leaders in function-based behavior support. Individuals from the work group are available on a limited basis to provide training at the request of school districts. Contact information is included in the Supplementary Section to this chapter. Alternatively, potential training resources include special education teachers, certified school psychologists, licensed clinical psychologists with behavioral training, behavioral specialists hired by the educational services district (or equivalent), and research teams at local universities.

Not all the individuals listed above will have experience or materials to conduct training in function-based behavior support. The school or school district should be prudent in making this decision. We recommend that schools should require the following characteristics in an individual hired to conduct FBA-BSP training with members of the individual behavior support team:

- Experience conducting FBAs.
- Experience designing and evaluating BSPs.
- Experience training teams to conduct FBA-BSP.
- Experience in general education settings.
- Available on a regular basis for at least 2 years for training, consultation, and support.
- Uses data-based decision making.
- Sensitive to practical realities of implementing FBA-BSP in schools.

The following is a brief summary of one training model. Each trainer will have his or her own approach and his or her own materials for training. However, many basic elements will be similar across trainers. Training can be conducted for the team members of one school or concurrently with multiple teams from multiple schools within a district. Training of multiple teams at once is, of course, much more cost-effective for a school district. The training model presented in this chapter assumes implementation at the school district level.

The conceptual framework for this training model can be described as a Learn–Implement–Train–Lead Model (based on Schmidt & Finnegan, 1993). In the "Learn" component, team members attend a series of comprehensive in-service workshops to learn about different aspects of the FBA-BSP process. The format of the training will vary depending on the preferences of the trainer and the school district. In some formats, the in-service workshops occur once a month and last a half-day. Each half-day workshop is dedicated to a different component of the FBA-BSP process. In other formats, 2–3 days are set aside for in-service workshops prior to the beginning of the school year. The team receives training in the entire FBA-BSP process within this condensed period of time.

In the "Implement" component, team members will implement the skills discussed during the workshop at their own school. In the Train–Lead component of the model, an individual from each team is chosen to become the school's FBA-BSP team leader/trainer. This person attends workshops to learn the skills to become a trainer. This is the "Train" component of the model. The team leader then implements the skills learned at his or her own school. This is the "Lead" component of the model.

The Learn–Implement training proceeds as follows: Participating team members are identified by each school. Each team comprises a representative sample of school staff as delineated in Chapter 6. Team members from all participating schools within a district meet in a central location for the series of in-service workshops (whether held once a month throughout the year, or for 2–3 days at the beginning of the year). This central location is often the district administration building. (A proposed budget should allocate funds to pay for substitutes so that team members may be released from their daily duties to attend these training sessions.) The training format that occurs over 2–3 full-day sessions before the school year begins (vs. several half-days over the course of a year) has two primary advantages:

1. The team members have been exposed to most of the FBA-BSP content and process prior to the beginning of the year. Thus, they can begin to work with one or two students and go through the process much faster than if they are learning skills piece by piece throughout the school year.
2. The team can be trained during staff development days that occur at the beginning of the school year rather than be taken out of their classrooms or away from their responsibilities throughout the school year.

At each session, the trainer leads a presentation and discussion of material covering the competencies listed above. Competencies are covered in enough detail to meet the needs of the participating schools. Competencies are sequenced so that each skill can be built upon another. Time should be allotted during these sessions for the teams to meet and plan how to implement the new material at their own schools. At each of these sessions, teams will develop an action plan for the upcoming month. In between sessions, the trainer should visit each school, observe the team members implementing new competencies, provide feedback, and consult with team members about obstacles that they encounter. By the end of the school year, each team member should be able to demonstrate mastery of each competency. The second half of the training sequence is Train and Lead. The major objective of this part of training is to ensure that schools can effectively implement individual behavior support without the assistance of an outside agency. One individual from each team is selected to become the FBA-BSP team leader at his or her school. This selection should be based on demonstration of (1) mastery of all of the necessary competencies, (2) interest in becoming a trainer, and (3) administrative support from their school principal. These trainers-in-training would attend in-service workshops and receive on-site coaching in order to learn the following competencies:

- Organizing the referral and intervention process within the school.
- Running an efficient, productive meeting.
- Designating roles and responsibilities.
- Facilitating and consulting with observers and interviewers.
- Training school personnel to conduct FBAs.
- Training school personnel to design, implement, and modify BSPs.
- Evaluating the FBA-BSP process.

The FBA-BSP consultant should observe the trainer-in-training at his or her school, provide feedback, and facilitate problem solving regarding any difficulties that arise. The Learn–Implement–Train–Lead Model is illustrated in Figure 8.1.

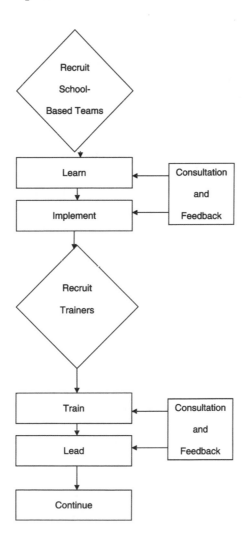

FIGURE 8.1. Training model.

LEADERSHIP MODELS

In Chapter 6, we outlined the roles that will need to be filled for each individual behavior support team: coordinator, referral liaison and behavioral expert. Each team may choose to use a different leadership model to fill these roles. The team's choice will be based on the school's resources, individual preferences, and the internal skill capacity of the school. Leadership within a team is often an evolutionary process. As the individual team members develop more skill in FBA-BSP, they are more likely to change from an individual-based to a team-based model of leadership. In the following section, we identify three possible leadership models and discuss the advantages and disadvantages of each.

Model 1

In the first model, the roles of coordinator, referral liaison, and behavioral expert are all served by the same person. This model may be common in a school that has little or no internal capacity for behavioral support. In this situation, the school is likely to contract for the services of an outside behavioral expert. This person is contacted about individual children with behavior problems, conducts the FBA, and develops a BSP. Team members may be included, but their participation is usually peripheral, limited to minimal input at the assessment and intervention phases. For a school that is in the initial stages of developing a system of individual behavior support, this may be the best place to start.

The primary advantage of this model is that one person is accountable for all activities related to FBA-BSP. Increased accountability may increase the likelihood that FBA-BSP tasks are completed in a timely manner. Additionally, the system is likely to be more organized. Without division of responsibility there is no opportunity for miscommunication among team members.

There are several limitations to this model:

1. In a school with a moderate to large number of students, one person will not be enough to serve the school's individual behavior support needs. The individual will have to spread his or her time so thin that he or she will not be able to do an adequate job with any individual student.

2. Relying on one person to manage individual problem behaviors tends to breed a sense of separation of responsibility from problem behavior. Problem behavior becomes "somebody else's problem."

3. The sustainability of the school's individual behavior support system becomes dependent on the continued employment of one person. There are a number of reasons why the behavioral consultant may be available to the school for only a limited time. For example, the consultant may choose another job, become ill, or financial support may run out. Individual behavior support is too

critical to a school's success to depend on the uncertainty of individual employment.

4. An outside consultant is unfamiliar with the day-to-day changes that occur within a school. Outside consultants are unaware of practical limitations within a school. They have less opportunity to foster the working relationships with teachers that are critical to the success of behavior support plan implementation.

5. Hiring an outside consultant can be quite costly.

6. An outside behavioral consultant can be difficult to reach or frequently unavailable to staff.

Model 2

In the second model, two individuals share most of the workload. The role of coordinator and referral liaison is filled by a member of the school staff, while someone with behavioral expertise conducts the FBAs and designs BSPs. In the initial stages of individual behavior support, the person with behavioral expertise is likely to be an outside behavioral consultant. However, as individuals from the school receive training in FBA-BSP and build internal capacity for doing FBA-BSP, the behavioral consultant may come from the school staff.

Because the work is divided between two people, this model may be more stable than the first model. In this model, the school would be better equipped to handle more referrals. The coordinator/referral liaison would be much more accessible to the school staff. As a result, the behavior support person would be more responsive to teacher requests for assistance. The advantages and limitations of hiring an outside behavior consultant apply to this model as well.

Model 3

The third model reflects a true team-based approach to individual behavior support. In this model, there are multiple individuals on the individual behavior support team with competency in FBA-BSP. These individuals share the workload on different Action Teams for different referrals. The coordinator/referral liaison is a within-building staff member. In this model, an outside behavior consultant is not necessary. This model can be achieved after a school has invested the time and resources to increase within-building capacity for FBA-BSP.

The major disadvantage to this approach is the increased likelihood of disorganization and miscommunication as responsibilities are shared across multiple individuals. In this model, the coordinator must be extremely efficient and organized.

This team-based approach has multiple advantages. Because the workload is shared by multiple individuals, the team can respond to more requests for assistance. Also, by sharing the workload, no one person should become over-whelmed. With a team-based approach, the school is more likely to feel respon-sible for managing problem behavior rather than thinking of problem behavior as someone else's domain. Because this model is more resilient to staff turnover, the individual behavior support system should be easier to sustain.

SUPPLEMENTARY SECTION

Contact Information for the Functional Assessment Work Group at the University of Oregon

Deanne Crone, PhD
5208 University of Oregon
Eugene, OR 97403
dcrone@oregon.uoregon.edu

Rob Horner, PhD
1761 Alder Street
University of Oregon
Eugene, OR 97403
robh@oregon.uoregon.edu

References on Schoolwide Discipline and Behavior Support (Compiled by George Sugai, PhD)

- Battistich, V., Watson, M., Solomon, D., Schaps, E., & Solomon, J. (1991). The Child Development Project: A comprehensive program for the development of prosocial character. In W. M. Kurtines & J. L. Gewirtz (Eds.), *Handbook of moral behavior and development, Vol. 3: Application* (pp. 1–34). Hillsdale, NJ: Erlbaum.
- Bear, G. G. (1990). Best practices in school discipline. In A. Thomas & J. Grimes (Eds.), *Best practices in school psychology* (Vol. 2, pp. 649–663). Washington, DC: National Association of School Psychologists.
- Colvin, G., Kameenui, E. J., & Sugai, G. (1993). School-wide and classroom management: Reconceptualizing the integration and management of students with behavior problems in general education. *Education and Treatment of Children, 16,* 361–381.
- Colvin, G., Sugai, G., Good, R. H., III, & Lee, Y. (1997). Using active supervision and precorrection to improve transition behaviors in an elementary school. *School Psychology Quarterly, 12,* 344–363.
- Colvin, G., Sugai, G., & Kameenui, E. (1994). *Curriculum for establishing a proactive schoolwide discipline plan.* Eugene: Project Prepare. Behavioral Research and Teaching, College of Education, University of Oregon.
- Gottfredson, D. C. (1987). An evaluation of an organization development approach to reducing school disorder. *Evaluation Review, 11,* 739–763.
- Gottfredson, D. C., Gottfredson, G. D., & Hybl, L. G. (1993). Managing adolescent be-

havior: A multiyear, multischool study. *American Educational Research Journal, 30*, 179–215.

- Gottfredson, D. C., Gottfredson, G. D., & Skroban, S. (1996). A multimodel school based prevention demonstration. *Journal of Adolescent Research, 11*, 97–115.
- Gottfredson, D. C., Karweit, N. L., & Gottfredson, G. D. (1989). *Reducing disorderly behavior in middle schools* (Report No. 47). Baltimore: Center of Research on Elementary and Middle Schools, Johns Hopkins University.
- Gresham, F. M., Sugai, G., Horner, R. H., Quinn, M. M., & McInerney, M. (1998). *Classroom and school-wide practices that support children's social competence: A synthesis of research.* Washington, DC: American Institutes of Research and Office of Special Education Programs.
- Hyman, I., Flanagan, D., & Smith, K. (1982). Discipline in the schools. In C. R. Reynolds & T. B. Gutkin (Eds.), *The handbook of school psychology* (pp. 454–480). New York: Wiley.
- Kazdin, A. E. (1982). Applying behavioral principles in the schools. In C. R. Reynolds & T. B. Gutkin (Eds.), *The handbook of school psychology* (pp. 501–529). New York: Wiley.
- Knoff, H. M. (1985). Best practices in dealing with discipline referrals. In A. Thomas & J. Grimes (Eds.), *Best practices in school psychology* (pp. 251–262). Washington, DC: National Association of School Psychologists.
- Lewis, T. J., & Sugai, G. (1999). Effective Behavior Support: A systems approach to proactive school-wide management. *Focus on Exceptional Children, 31*(6), 1–24.
- Lewis-Palmer, T., Sugai, G., & Larson, S. (1999). Using data to guide decisions about program implementation and effectiveness. *Effective School Practices, 17*(4), 47–53.
- Martens, B. K., Peterson, R. L., Witt, J. C., & Cirone, S. (1986). Teacher perceptions of school-based interventions. *Exceptional Children, 53*, 213–223.
- Mayer, G. R. (1999). Constructive discipline for school personnel. *Education and Treatment of Children, 22*, 36–54.
- Mayer, G. R., & Butterworth, T. (1979). A preventive approach to school violence and vandalism: An experimental study. *Personnel and Guidance Journal, 57*, 436–441.
- Mayer, G. R., Butterworth, T., Komoto, T., & Benoit, R. (1983). The influence of the school principal on the consultant's effectiveness. *Elementary School Guidance and Counseling, 17*, 274–279.
- Mayer, G. R., Butterworth, T., Nafpaktitis, M., & Suzer-Azaroff, B. (1983). Preventing school vandalism and improving discipline: A three year study. *Journal of Applied Behavior Analysis, 16*, 355–369.
- Short, P. M., & Short, R. J. (1987). Beyond technique: Personal and organizational influences on school discipline. *High School Journal, 71*(1), 31–36.
- Strein, W. (1988). Classroom-based elementary school affective education programs: A critical review. *Psychology in the Schools, 25*, 288–296.
- Sugai, G., & Horner, R. H. (1999). Discipline and behavioral support: Preferred processes and practices. *Effective School Practices, 17*(4), 10–22.
- Sugai, G., & Pruitt, R. (1993). *Phases, steps, and guidelines for building schoolwide behavior management programs: A practitioner's handbook* (Behavior Disorders Handbook No. 1). Eugene: Behavior Disorders Program, University of Oregon.

- Sulzer-Azaroff, B., & Mayer, G. R. (1986). *Achieving educational excellence: Using behavioral strategies.* New York: Holt, Rinehart & Winston.
- Sulzer-Azaroff, B., & Mayer, G. R. (1994). *Achieving educational excellence: Behavior analysis for achieving classroom and schoolwide behavior change.* San Marcos, CA: Western Image.
- Taylor-Greene, S., Brown, D., Nelson, L., Longton, J., Gassman, T., Cohen, J., Swartz, J., Horner, R. H., Sugai, G., & Hall, S. (1997). School-wide behavioral support: Starting the year off right. *Journal of Behavioral Education, 7,* 99–112.
- Todd, A. W., Horner, R. H., Sugai, G., & Colvin, G. (1999). Individualizing schoolwide discipline for students with chronic problem behaviors: A team approach. *Effective School Practices, 17*(4), 72–82.
- Todd, A. W., Horner, R. H., Sugai, G., & Sprague, J. R. (1999). Effective behavior support: Strengthening schoolwide systems through a team-based approach. *Effective School Practices, 17*(4), 23–27.
- Weissberg, R. P., Caplan, M. Z., & Sivo, P. J. (1989). A new conceptual framework for establishing school-based social competence promotion programs. In L. A. Bond & B. E. Compas (Eds.), *Primary prevention and promotion in the schools* (pp. 255–296). Newbury Park, CA: Sage.

Appendices

Request for Assistance Form

Date _____   Teacher/Team _____

                              IEP: Yes No (Circle)

Student Name _____ Grade _____

Situations	Problem Behaviors	Most Common Result
What have you tried/used? How has it worked?		

What is your behavioral goal/expectation for this student? _____

What have you tried to date to change the situations in which the problem behavior(s) occur?

__ Modified assignments to match the student's skills	__ Changed seating assignments	__ Changed schedule of activities	Other?
__ Arranged tutoring to improve the student's academic skills	__ Changed curriculum	__ Provided extra assistance	

What have you tried to date to teach expected behaviors?

__ Reminders about expected behavior when problem behavior is likely	__ Clarified rules and expected behavior for the whole class	__ Practiced the expected behaviors in class	Other?
__ Reward program for expected behavior	__ Oral agreement with the student	__ Self-management program	
__ Systematic feedback about behavior	__ Individual written contract with the student	__ Contract with student/ with parents	

What consequences have you tried to date for the problem behavior?

__ Loss of privileges	__ Note or phone call to the student's parents	__ Office referral	Other?
__ Time-out	__ Detention	__ Reprimand	
__ Referral to school counselor	__ Meeting with the student's parents	__ Individual meeting with the student	

(continued)

APPENDIX A. Request for Assistance Form (page 2 of 2)

WHEN ADDRESSING THIS PROBLEM, PLEASE CONSIDER THE FOLLOWING QUESTIONS:

1. When is the problem behavior(s) *most* and *least* likely to occur?
   - On particular days of the week (e.g., Monday) or times of day (e.g., right after recess)?
   - During or after interactions with certain people (e.g., during small, cooperative group projects)?
   - During certain types of activity or tasks (e.g., during apparently difficult or boring work)?
   - In connection with particular features of the physical environment (e.g., noisy, crowded)?
   - Features of routine (e.g., when there are unexpected changes or when a preferred activity is canceled)?
   - Medical or physical factors (e.g., apparent hunger or lack of sleep)?
   - Other influences?
2. What do you think the student(s) may gain from the problem behaviors?
   - Attention? What kind of attention? From whom?
   - Avoid an apparently difficult or boring activity?
   - Avoid teacher interaction?
   - Get control of a situation?
   - Avoid embarrassment in front of peers?

Summary of Behavior

Setting Events & Predictors	Behaviors of Concern	Maintaining Consequences

3. Are there appropriate behaviors that the student could use that would make the problem behavior unnecessary?
4. Teacher support team decision
   - ❑ Some suggestions regarding interventions to try.
   - ❑ Referral to a different team for assessment (speech hearing, academic): _____
   - ❑ Formation of an action team to conduct a functional assessment and develop a plan of support.
5. Date for follow-up _____

Functional Behavioral Assessment–Behavior Support Plan Protocol (F-BSP Protocol)

FUNCTIONAL BEHAVIORAL ASSESSMENT INTERVIEW—TEACHER/STAFF/PARENT

Student Name: _____ Age: ____ Grade: ____ Date: _____

Person(s) interviewed: _____

Interviewer: _____

Student Profile: What is the student good at or what are some strengths that the student brings to school?

_____

_____

Step 1A: Interview Teacher/Staff/Parent

Description of the Behavior

What does the problem behavior(s) look like?
How often does the problem behavior(s) occur?
How long does the problem behavior(s) last when it does occur?
How disruptive or dangerous is the problem behavior(s)?

Description of the Antecedent
Identifying Routines: When, where, and with whom are problem behaviors most likely?

Schedule (Times)	Activity	Specific Problem Behavior	Likelihood of Problem Behavior	With Whom Does Problem Occur?
			Low High 1 2 3 4 5 6	
			1 2 3 4 5 6	
			1 2 3 4 5 6	
			1 2 3 4 5 6	
			1 2 3 4 5 6	
			1 2 3 4 5 6	
			1 2 3 4 5 6	
			1 2 3 4 5 6	

(continued)

Summarize Antecedent (and Setting Events)

What situations seem to set off the problem behavior? (difficult tasks, transitions, structured activities, small-group settings, teacher's request, particular individuals, etc.) **When is the problem behavior most likely to occur?** (times of day and days of the week) **When is the problem behavior least likely to occur?** (times of day and days of the week) **Setting Events: Are there specific conditions, events, or activities that make the problem behavior worse?** (missed medication, history of academic failure, conflict at home, missed meals, lack of sleep, history of problems with peers, etc.)

Description of the Consequence

What usually happens after the behavior occurs? (what is the teacher's reaction, how do other students react, is the student sent to the office, does the student get out of doing work, does the student get in a power struggle, etc.)

- - - - - - End of Interview - - - - - -

Step 2A: Propose a Testable Explanation

Setting Event	Antecedent	Behavior	Consequence
		1.	
		2.	

Function of the Behavior

For each ABC sequence listed above, why do you think the behavior is occurring? (to get teacher attention, to get peer attention, gets desired object/activity, escapes undesirable activity, escapes demand, escapes particular people, etc.)

1. _____

2. _____

How confident are you that your testable explanation is accurate?

Very sure			So-so		Not at all sure
6	5	4	3	2	1

(continued)

FUNCTIONAL BEHAVIORAL ASSESSMENT INTERVIEW—STUDENT

Student Name: _____ **Age:** ____ **Grade:** ____ **Date:** _____
Interviewer: _____

Student Profile: What are the things you like to do, or do well, while at school? (activities, classes, helping others, etc.)

_____
_____

Step 1B: Interview Student

Description of the Behavior

What are some things you do that get you in trouble or that are a problem at school? (talking out, not getting work done, fighting, etc.)
How often do you _____**?** (Insert the behavior listed by the student)
How long does _____ **usually last each time it happens?**
How serious is _____**?** (Do you or another student end up getting hurt? Are other students distracted?)

Description of the Antecedent
Identifying Routines: When, where, and with whom are problem behaviors most likely?

Schedule (Times)	Activity	Specific Problem Behavior	Likelihood of Problem Behavior	With Whom Does Problem Occur?
			Low High 1 2 3 4 5 6	
			1 2 3 4 5 6	
			1 2 3 4 5 6	
			1 2 3 4 5 6	
			1 2 3 4 5 6	
			1 2 3 4 5 6	
			1 2 3 4 5 6	
			1 2 3 4 5 6	
			1 2 3 4 5 6	

(continued)

131

Summarize Antecedent (and Setting Events)

What kind of things make it more likely that you will have this problem? (difficult tasks, transitions, structured activities, small-group settings, teacher's request, particular individuals, etc.)   **When and where is the problem most likely to happen?** (days of week, specific classes, hallways, bathrooms)   **When is the problem behavior least likely to occur?** (days of week, specific classes, hallways, bathrooms)   **Setting Events: Is there there anything that happens before or after school or in between classes that makes it more likely that you'll have a problem?** (missed medication, history of academic failure, conflict at home, missed meals, lack of sleep, history of problems with peers, etc.)

Description of the Consequence

What usually happens after the problem occurs? (what is the teacher's reaction, how do other students react, is the student sent to the office, does the student get out of doing work, does the student get in a power struggle, etc.)

- - - - - - End of Interview - - - - - -

Step 2B: Develop a Testable Explanation

Setting Event	Antecedent	Behavior	Consequence
		1.	
		2.	
		3.	

Function of the Behavior

For each ABC sequence listed above, why do you think the behavior is occurring? (to get teacher attention, to get peer attention, gets desired object/activity, escapes undesirable activity, escapes demand, escapes particular people, etc.)

1. _____

2. _____

3. _____

(continued)

Step 3: Rate Your Confidence in the Testable Explanation

If you completed both interviews, was there agreement on these parts? (Y/N)
(a) Setting Events _____ (b) Antecedents _____ (c) Behaviors _____ (d) Consequences _____
(e) Function _____

How confident are you that your testable explanation is accurate?

Very sure			So-so		Not at all sure
6	5	4	3	2	1

Step 4: Conduct Observations (If Necessary)

- If student has an identified disability and is at risk of suspension, expulsion, or change in placement you must conduct an observation of student.
- If student does not meet above criteria, but confidence rating is 1, 2, 3, or 4, you should conduct observations to better understand when, where, and why the problem behavior is occurring.
- If student does not meet above criteria, and confidence rating is 5 or 6, you may go directly to Step 6

Summarize Observation Data

Setting Event	Antecedent	Behavior	Consequence
		1.	
		2.	
		3.	

Function of the Behavior

For each ABC sequence listed above, why do you think the behavior is occurring? (to get teacher attention, to get peer attention, gets desired object/activity, escapes undesirable activity, escapes demand, escapes particular people, etc.)

1. _____

2. _____

3. _____

Step 5: Confirm/Modify Testable Explanation

Was there agreement between the teacher interview and the observation? Y/N

a) Setting Events _____ (b) Antecedents _____ (c) Behaviors _____ (d) Consequences _____ (e) Function _____

Was there agreement between the student interview and the observation? Y/N

a) Setting Events _____ (b) Antecedents _____ (c) Behaviors _____ (d) Consequences _____ (e) Function _____

Based on the interviews and observations, what is your working testable explanation for why the problem behavior occurs?

_____

_____

(continued)

Step 6: Build a Competing Behavior Pathway

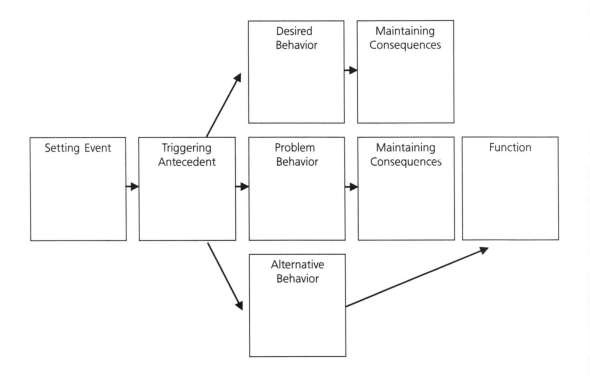

Setting Event Strategies	Antecedent Strategies	Behavior Teaching Strategies	Consequence Strategies

(continued)

Step 7: Select Intervention Strategies

Tasks	Person Responsible	By When	Review Date	Evaluation Decision • Monitor • Modify • Discontinue

*If emergency behavior management procedures are necessary, attach crisis plan as separate sheet.

(continued)

Step 8: Evaluate Plan

Behavioral Goal (use specific, observable, measurable descriptions of goal)

What is the short-term behavioral goal?

_____ Expected date

What is the long-term behavioral goal?

_____ Expected date

Evaluation Procedures

Data to Be Collected	Procedures for Data Collection	Person Responsible	Timeline

Plan review date: _____

We agree to the conditions of this plan:

Student	(date)	Parent or guardian	(date)
Teacher	(date)	Teacher	(date)
Action Team member	(date)	Action Team member	(date)

(continued)

136

INSTRUCTIONS FOR COMPLETING THE FUNCTIONAL BEHAVIORAL ASSESSMENT—BEHAVIOR SUPPORT PLAN PROTOCOL (F-BSP PROTOCOL)

The F-BSP Protocol was designed as a tool to guide the process of completing a functional behavioral assessment (FBA) and of linking the assessment to the design of an individual behavior support plan (BSP). The F-BSP Protocol is divided into eight Steps: (1) Interview Teacher/Staff/Parent/Student; (2) Propose a Testable Explanation; (3) Rate Your Confidence in the Testable Explanation; (4) Conduct Observations; (5) Confirm/Modify Testable Explanation; (6) Build a Competing Behavior Pathway; (7) Select Intervention Strategies; and (8) Evaluation Plan.

The F-BSP Protocol can be used to complete either a simple FBA or a full FBA. In a simple FBA, Steps 4 and 5 are omitted. The Student Interview portion of Step 1 is omitted as well in a simple FBA.

Demographic Information

Before any interview, it is important to explain the purpose of the interview to the interviewee. Spend a little time explaining why you are doing the interview, indicate that you think it will take about 20–30 minutes to complete, and note that you will follow up with the interviewee once the FBA is completed.

Take a few minutes to complete the demographic information at the top of page 1. For confidentiality purposes, you may choose to use only the student's initials or to identify the student by his or her student number.

In the space next to "Person(s) Interviewed," indicate the person's relationship to the student, (math teacher, lunchroom monitor, parent, etc). In the space next to "Interviewer," indicate the interviewer's role in the behavior support process (Action Team member, team leader, school psychologist, etc.).

In the space next to "Student Profile," ask the interviewee to list some of the student's strengths, skills, or talents. Also list items or activities that the student enjoys or will work for. This information will help you to design a BSP that builds on the student's strengths and that includes consequences that are personally reinforcing to the student.

Step 1A: Interview Teacher/Staff/Parent

The purpose of Step 1 is to get a clear understanding of the problem behavior(s) of concern and to identify routines that predict or support the problem behavior. This is accomplished by generating a clear definition of the problem behavior, and by identifying the setting events, antecedents, and consequences of the problem behavior.

The first interview should be conducted with the person who made the initial request for assistance. This may be the student's primary teacher or any other adult with whom the student has significant contact (e.g., the lunchroom monitor, school counselor, or algebra teacher). A simple FBA typically includes only one teacher interview. A full FBA may include additional interviews with relevant adults, including other teachers or a parent. Copies of the teacher/staff/parent interview can be made to accommodate the need for multiple interviews.

(continued)

Description of the Behavior

The interviewer asks the interviewee four questions regarding the problem behavior.

1. What does the problem behavior(s) look like?
2. How often does the problem behavior(s) occur?
3. How long does the problem behavior(s) last when it does occur?
4. How disruptive or dangerous is the problem behavior?

Write down the answers to each question in the space provided. Prompt the interviewee to be as specific as possible. If the answer to the question is not specific, measurable, or observable, prompt the interviewee to be clearer in his or her response. For example, in response to question 1, the interviewee may say *"Marisa is spacey and distractible in class."* This definition of the problem behavior is unclear—"spacey and distractible" may mean something different to the interviewer than it does to the interviewee. Prompt the interviewee by saying, *"How do you know when Marisa is being spacey and distractible? What does it look like?"* Continue to prompt the interviewee until the description of the problem behavior is clear enough that two observers would be able to recognize it independently. If the interviewee describes more than one problem behavior in question 1, be sure to get answers to questions 2, 3, and 4 for each problem behavior. Make a clear note of this on the interview form.

Description of the Antecedent

An *antecedent* is an event or circumstance that happens before a behavior occurs. It can be thought of as the predictor of a problem behavior. Examples of antecedents that could set off problem behavior include asking the student to do a demanding or long task; placing the student next to another child whom he dislikes; or expecting a child to complete a task during unstructured work time. The same antecedent could set off problem behavior for one student, while it helps another student to perform successfully. Because antecedents can vary so much between different students, it is very important to understand the antecedents that matter to the student with whom you are concerned. You can begin to identify the antecedents to problem behavior by looking at the student's daily routine.

Begin by completing the table on the bottom of page 1. In the first two columns, fill in the student's daily schedule. In the first column, indicate the time period for the activity, and in the second column briefly describe the activity. For example, for a middle school student, you would write down the time for first period and the name of the class that the student has during first period. Then you would continue on through the last period of the day. The schedule for an elementary school student can be obtained from the student's primary teacher. An elementary school schedule is usually broken into smaller time periods, by subject or activity (e.g., math, science, circle time, etc.). The interview will go quicker if you can get the child's schedule and complete this section before you begin the interview. If you are interviewing a parent, you will complete the first two columns of this table a little differently. Ask the parent to think of the times of their day that are related to school. Some examples include getting ready for school in the morning, transportation to school, transportation home from school, and doing homework. Include all of these activities in the "Activity" column. Ask the parent to provide you with a general idea of times when these activities occur.

Complete the rest of the table for the time periods you have listed. Look at the first time period. Ask the interviewee if the student engages in problem behavior during that time period. If he or she does, ask the interviewee what type of problem behavior occurs. Write this down in the column marked "Specific Problem Behavior." The problem behaviors that you write down should reflect the problem behaviors that you discussed in the first section of the interview. You should already have a good description of these behaviors, so it is fine to write a brief description in this column (e.g., you could write "temper tantrum," "fighting," or "distractible" because these behaviors are specifically described in the first section).

(continued)

After you have written down the type of problem behavior that occurs during a time period, ask the interviewee how likely it is that the problem behavior will occur during that time period. Ask him or her to rate the likelihood on a scale of 1 to 6 where 1 means that it rarely happens and 6 means that it happens on a daily basis. Circle that number in the next column.

Finally, ask the interviewee with whom the problem is most likely to occur. Does the student get into trouble with other students? Is the student defiant toward the teacher? Perhaps the problem does not impact anyone other than the student. In this column, indicate if the problem occurs with peers, teacher, self, parent, or another significant person. If the interviewee indicates that the problem typically occurs with specific peers, you should indicate these students by using their initials only. Complete each of these columns for each time period listed.

Summarize Antecedent (and Setting Events)

The next section helps you to summarize and clarify the information you have learned from the description of the student's schedule. In this section, the interviewee will answer four questions:

1. What situations seem to set off the problem behavior?
2. When is the problem behavior most likely to occur?
3. When is the problem behavior least likely to occur?
4. Are there specific conditions, events, or activities that make the problem behavior worse?

To answer the first question, take a look at the completed table with the interviewee. First look at the times when the student is most likely to engage in problem behavior—times when the likelihood is rated a 4, 5, or 6. Is there anything similar about those times? For example, is each time period an unstructured time, or do each of the time periods require the student to do demanding work on his or her own? Perhaps each is a time when the student's sibling is in the same class. Try to determine what is similar about the problematic routines that tend to set off the problem behavior. If the interviewee has trouble answering this question, prompt him or her by saying, *"If you wanted to make the problem behavior occur, what would you do?"*

Ask the interviewee what times of the day and days of the week the problem behavior is most likely to occur. If his or her answer is different than what you would expect (based on the information given in the schedule table), ask the interviewee to clarify his or her answer.

Ask the interviewee when the problem behavior is least likely to occur. Knowing when the problem behavior does not occur can help you identify things that work for the student. That is, there are some routines when the student does not get into trouble. If you can identify what it is about those routines that helps the student be successful, you can better determine how to change the student's unsuccessful routines.

Setting events are situations or circumstances that make it more likely that a problem behavior will occur or that make the problem behavior more intense. Some examples include: if the student has a fight with a parent right before coming to school, if the student didn't get enough sleep or missed a meal, or if the student misses taking medication. Ask the interviewee if he or she knows of certain situations that tend to make the student's problem behavior worse, or more likely to occur.

Description of the Consequence

In this section, you want to find out what usually happens after the problem behavior occurs. Is the student ignored or do all of his peers start to laugh? Is the student sent to the office? Is the student sent to time-out? Ask the interviewee what typically happens after the problem behavior occurs and what impact those consequences seem to have on the problem behavior. In other words, do the consequences make the problem behavior stop, improve, or get worse?

(continued)

End of Interview

At this point, the face-to-face portion of the interview is completed. Next you will summarize the information you have learned from the interview to create a "testable explanation" of why the problem behavior is occurring.

If you need to interview additional teachers or other adults (including parents), make copies of the first two pages of the F-BSP protocol and use the copies for as many interviews as you plan to conduct.

Step 2A: Propose a Testable Explanation

ABC Sequence

A testable explanation is one of the most important pieces of the F-BSP process. It is the summary of everything you have learned about the problem behavior and the link to designing an effective, relevant BSP.

Begin to build your testable hypothesis by listing the problem behavior. It is likely that a student will engage in more than one type of problem behavior. For example, the same student might fight with other students and refuse to follow teacher directions. List each *type* of problem behavior separately in the column labeled "Behavior." (Don't list every single problem behavior displayed. E.g., if fighting consists of pushing, hitting, and yelling at other students, you would lump all three behaviors into one *type* of behavior: "fighting.")

Next, for each type of behavior you have listed, indicate the antecedents that tend to set off or predict that behavior. List them under the column headed "Antecedents." Refer back to the interview information to identify the antecedents.

For each type of behavior you have listed, indicate the consequences that tend to support the problem behavior in the "Consequences" column. The interviewee will have told you about many potential consequences that occur. List the ones that seem to make the behavior continue or worsen. For example, a student who makes inappropriate jokes in class might encounter two consequences. First, the joke might be ignored by other students and he is unlikely to tell that joke again. Second, he might get a lot of attention and laughter over his inappropriate joke. In that case, he is likely to tell other inappropriate jokes or tell the same joke in other classes. In this example, the ignoring consequence did not support the problem behavior, but the attention/laughter consequence did. For your testable explanation of why the problem behavior is occurring, you want to list the consequences that support the problem behavior. In the example, you would write "peer attention and laughter" under the column that is headed "Consequences."

Finally, if there are any setting events that make the problem behavior worse or more likely to occur, list them under the column headed "Setting Event."

Complete the Setting Event, Antecedent, and Consequence boxes for each *type* of behavior that you have listed. Each set of these is called an *ABC sequence*.

Function of the Behavior

For each ABC sequence, you want to determine why you think the behavior is occurring. At this point you can describe the behavior, you know what situations set it off, and you know what consequences make it continue or get worse. But why is the behavior happening? What function does it serve for the student? Some common functions include: to get peer attention, to get adult attention, to get out of doing difficult work, or to get away from someone the student doesn't like. For each ABC sequence, decide what you think is really motivating the problem behavior and write it down in the space provided.

Once you become more familiar with the F-BSP Protocol, it will become fairly easy to complete Step 2. At that point, we suggest that you complete Step 2 with the interviewee to check for his or her agreement with your summary of the interview.

(continued)

Step 1B: Interview Student

The student interview follows the same format as the teacher/staff/parent interview. The wording of some of the questions has been changed to be more appropriate for talking with a student, but they result in the same type of information.

We have found that the student interview is most useful when used with a student in third grade or higher. Younger students typically lack the awareness of their own behavior that is necessary to provide informative answers to the interview questions. However, younger students are able to respond to the Student Profile question, "What are things that you like to do, or do well, while at school?" It is important to ask every student this question. The answer to the question will give you information about the objects or activities that are personally meaningful to the student. For example, the student may prefer using the computer to going to gym class. Once you have an idea of what is personally meaningful for the student, you can build it into the student's BSP. For example, the student could earn extra time to use the computer by meeting her behavioral goals.

It is very important to make the student feel comfortable during the interview process. It is helpful if the student is already familiar with the interviewer. The interview should take place in a setting that is comfortable for the student. For example, a younger child will be less comfortable sitting in an adult-sized chair at an adult-sized table than he or she would be sitting at a student-sized desk. In addition, a student who is frequently called down to the principal's office for discipline issues will be uncomfortable being interviewed in the principal's office. Choose a neutral setting, such as an empty classroom, the counselor's office, or a family resource room. To maintain student confidentiality, any interview (including the teacher and parent interviews) should be conducted in private.

Be careful to clearly explain the purpose of the interview to the student. Also, make sure the student understands that he or she is not in trouble and will not get in trouble for answering the interviewer's questions. It is also helpful to let the student know that his or her parents have given permission for the student to participate in the interview.

The following script may be helpful in introducing the purpose of the interview to the student:

Hi _____. I'm _____. I am (a teacher, school counselor, etc.) at this school.

One of the things I do is work with kids who are having a hard time in school. I try to figure out how to help them do better in school so they can like school better. I think one of the best ways to do that is to talk to the kids and find out what they think is good and bad about school

So, I'd like to ask you some questions. I'd like to find out what you like about school and what are some of the things that get you into trouble at school. Is that okay?

If I ask you a question that you don't understand, just say "I don't understand" and I'll try to explain it. Okay?

There's one more thing I want to tell you. I want to be able to remember what you told me so we can figure out how to help you do well in school. I can remember better when I write things down, so I'm going to write your answers down on this piece of paper.

Okay, let's get started.

Step 2B: Propose a Testable Explanation

This is the same process you follow after completing the teacher/staff/parent interview. Refer to Step 2A for more information.

Step 3: Rate Your Confidence in the Testable Explanation

Before going further in the F-BSP process, you want to assess how confident you are that you understand the problem behavior and why it is occurring. The best way to do this is to compare the sources of information that you have collected.

(continued)

At this point, you have collected multiple interviews. The box under Step 3 provides you with space to compare the results of these interviews. Look at the testable explanations that you have generated after each interview. Overall, does it seem like the different interviews have generated the same information? Is there agreement between interviews on the setting events, antecedents, behaviors, consequences, and functions? After each item, write a "Y" for Yes there is agreement between interviews or a "N" for No if the interviews disagree. The more agreement you have between multiple sources, the more confident you can be in your testable explanation of the problem.

Next, the team should rate their confidence in the testable explanation. Indicate on a scale of 1 to 6 (1 = not at all confident, 6 = very sure) how confident the team is that they understand why the behavior is occurring, and under what circumstances. A score of 1, 2, 3, or 4 indicates that the team is not very confident in their understanding of the behavior and that they need additional information (usually observations in the classroom) before going on to develop a BSP.

Step 4: Conduct Observations

There are certain circumstances under which you are required to conduct an observation while doing a FBA and other circumstances when it is recommended. These circumstances are listed directly on the F-BSP Protocol.

If observations are warranted and conducted, summarize the observation data under Step 4. Once again, your purpose is to generate a testable explanation that lists the problem behavior, its setting events, antecedents, consequences, and functions. Follow the same format as discussed under Step 1: Interview Teacher/Staff/Parent.

Step 5: Confirm/Modify Testable Explanation

Observations of the student in a natural setting (classroom, playground, etc.) give you a clearer picture of the behavior described by the student, the teachers, and the parents. By supplementing the interview information with direct observations, you can confirm or modify your original testable explanation and settle on a working testable explanation. You will use this working testable explanation to build your BSP.

First compare the teacher interview with the observation. Was there agreement between the two sources of information on setting events, antecedents, behaviors, consequences, and functions? Mark a "Y" or "N" after each space. Compare the parent interview and student interview with the observation following the same method.

Now that you have compiled all of this information, what is your final working explanation for the problem behavior? Record your working explanation under the final question in Step 5.

Step 6: Build a Competing Behavior Pathway

If you have identified several different *types* of problem behavior, you will have a different testable explanation for each problem behavior. You will also need to build a separate competing behavior pathway for each type of problem behavior. Make copies of this page of the F-BSP Protocol as necessary.

Begin by recording your testable working explanation. In the box marked "Problem Behavior," write the type of problem behavior exhibited by the student. Next fill in the boxes for the "Setting Event," "Antecedent," and "Consequences" for that problem behavior. Finally, to the right of the box marked "Consequence," indicate the function of the problem behavior.

Next you must decide on the desired behavior and an acceptable, alternative behavior. The desired behavior can be thought of as the long-term goal. How do you hope this problem behavior will change in the long term? For example, if the problem behavior is that the student cries and rips up his paper when he thinks an assignment is too difficult, the desired behavior might be that the student is able to work quietly and complete independent seatwork. The acceptable alternative behavior can be thought of as a short-

(continued)

term goal. It is an improvement on the problem behavior in that it is more acceptable in the classroom. However, it is considered a short-term goal because, often, it is not possible to sustain over a long period of time. For example, an acceptable alternative behavior for this student might be to raise his hand and receive teacher assistance every time he encounters a problem he doesn't understand. It is critical that the alternative behavior serves the same function for the student that the problem behavior served. This provides the incentive for the student to begin to change his behavior. In the above example, if the student cries and rips up his paper to receive adult attention, then the acceptable alternative behavior is likely to be effective in producing a change in the student's behavior. It is an acceptable, more efficient way for the student to receive attention. However, if the student is crying and ripping up his paper to get out of doing the work, then the alternative behavior is likely to actually *worsen* his behavior. The alternative behavior is likely to bring more emphasis on completing the work rather than escaping it. Determining effective alternative behaviors is often a difficult challenge. It will take some time to gain mastery of this concept.

The next step is to begin to brainstorm strategies that will change the student's problem behavior. The Competing Behavior Pathway serves as a guide. Remember, the Competing Behavior Pathway tells you what the problem behavior is and what you would like the behavior to be. It also tells you how you can predict when the behavior will occur and what type of consequences tend to support, rather than reduce, the problem behavior. Each of these pieces gives you something to work with, something to change. A change in the sequence will bring about a change in the behavior. Include the student's teacher, parent, or other significant adults in this discussion. These individuals know the student well and will be able to suggest creative and individualized ideas for behavior change.

The table underneath the Competing Behavior Pathway lists Setting Event Strategies, Antecedent Strategies, Behavior Teaching Strategies, and Consequence Strategies. Underneath each heading you will list suggestions for changing and improving that part of the problem behavior sequence.

Begin by looking at the boxes for problem behavior, desired behavior, and alternative behavior. In order to change a problem behavior to the desired or alternative behaviors, you will need to teach the student how to perform those behaviors. Identify the skills that the student needs to perform the preferred behaviors. One of the strategies you should list is to teach those behaviors to the student.

A very powerful method for changing behavior is to clearly *define* the behavioral expectations, *teach* behavioral expectations, and then *reward* the student for following the behavioral expectations. Defining expectations is an antecedent strategy, teaching behavioral expectations is a behavior strategy, and rewarding expectations is a consequence strategy. Rewarding the student should be based on what you learned from the student in terms of what he or she enjoys at school. For example, if the student loves art, but hates to use the computer, you would suggest that he or she could earn a few extra minutes of art time for appropriate behavior rather than a few extra minutes of computer time.

As you brainstorm strategies for each column, try to individualize them to the student as much as possible. For example, if a setting event for problem behavior is that the student often misses breakfast, one suggestion would be to provide breakfast for the student at school. If a predictor for problem behavior is that the student acts out when he is seated next to a particular classmate, the antecedent strategy would be to separate the two students. As you can see, these strategies can be, and often are, very simple.

Brainstorm as many strategies as you can. You will not use them all. However, it is helpful to have a range of options to choose from. Also, if you implement some strategies and your plan is ineffective, you can come back to this page and you will have a "bank" of ideas to start with. You won't have to go back to the drawing board.

Step 7: Select Intervention Strategies

The next step is to choose the strategies that you are going to begin with. At this point, you have a large number of options to choose from, and you need to narrow it down to the optimal, initial strategies. It is critical that the student's teacher and parent (or whichever adult is most likely to implement the

(continued)

intervention strategies) are involved in this discussion. You cannot choose which strategies will work best without knowing the implementer's values, willingness, and ability to implement those strategies.

Begin with a reasonable number of intervention strategies. This number will vary depending on the problem addressed and the resources available. However, the people involved in implementing the interventions should be able to tell you what they can handle and what will put a strain on them. Remember, you are trying to get the biggest impact with the most efficient effort.

Choose strategies that will fit well within the context in which they are implemented. Choose strategies that will fit well with the teachers' and parents' values and attitudes toward behavior change.

Once you have chosen which strategies to implement, list them individually under the column labeled "Tasks." Sometimes you will have to break a task into several different parts in order to accomplish it. For example, if the task is to use a behavior card to monitor and reward the student's behavior, you might have to break it into the following parts: (1) Decide on the behavioral goals; (2) Create a behavior card; (3) Teach the student to use the behavior card; (4) Explain the behavior card system to the student's teachers and parents; (5) Decide how the student's appropriate behavior will be rewarded; (6) Decide who will be in charge of rewarding the student. Each of these parts are critical to accomplishing the original task.

After each task and its corresponding parts are listed, a person needs to be assigned responsibility for completing those tasks. Think about individuals' natural roles in the school and assign tasks accordingly. For example, if the task is to teach the student anger management skills and the school counselor teaches an anger management group, then the school counselor should be assigned that task. If the task is to modify the student's assignments, the teacher should be assigned that task. In addition to assigning a person to be responsible for each task, a deadline for implementation should also be assigned. That is, the group should decide how soon each task should begin. Also indicate the date by which the effectiveness of the strategy will be reviewed. It is a good idea to review a new intervention plan within 2 weeks of implementation.

This sheet is kept as a running record of the student's BSP. The next time that the team meets, they should review this page. First they should determine if the strategies were implemented as planned and the extent to which the strategies are working. These decisions should be based on evaluation data and teacher/parent/student feedback. After reviewing the effectiveness of each strategy, decide whether or not the strategy should continue to be monitored, should be modified, or should be discontinued. Write "Monitor," "Modify," or "Discontinue" in the space next to each strategy. If a strategy is to be modified, or if a new strategy is added, these changes should be added under the column labeled "Tasks." Once again, assign someone to be responsible for implementing the strategy, by a specific deadline, and with a specific review date.

Step 8: Evaluate Plan

The final step is to design a plan to evaluate the effect of the BSP on the student's behavior. Begin by identifying the short- and long-term goals. Remember that you identified short- and long-term goals when you identified the desired behavior and acceptable alternative behavior for the Competing Behavior Pathway. Write these short- and long-term goals on the evaluation plan. Try to be as specific as possible with your goals so that it is easy to determine if the goals have been met. For example, if one of the goals is to increase rate of homework completion, be specific about how frequently you expect the child to turn in homework for a short-term and a long-term goal. If the student is currently turning in 0% of his homework, your short-term goal might be to have him turn in 30% of his homework, while your long-term goal might be to have him turn in 80% of his homework. The more specific you are in writing your goal, the easier it will be to objectively decide if the student has met the goal. Once you have decided on short- and long-term goals, determine a date by which you expect the student to achieve those goals. Determine this date in conjunction with the teacher and parents of the student.

To determine if the goals have been met, you will need to collect data on the student's performance. The data collected will differ depending on the behavior support strategy and the goal. For example, the

(continued)

student may be placed on a behavior card and his goal may be to earn 80% of his points on a daily basis. In this example, the data collected is the points on the behavior card and the procedures for collecting data is the behavior card itself. As another example, if the student's goal is to reduce the number of times he fights with other students in class, the teacher might keep a frequency count of the number of fights observed. In this example, the data collected is the number of fights, and the procedure for data collection is the teacher keeping a frequency count. For each goal, you will need to determine the type of data to be collected and a procedure for collecting that data. It is also critical to assign someone to be responsible for collecting the data and indicate the timeline for beginning and reviewing the data.

Agreement of All Key Individuals

Finally, all of the key individuals in this process should sign the last page. Their signature indicates that they understand the assessment information, the BSP, and the evaluation plan. Their signatures also indicate that they agree to implement any responsibility that was assigned to them. Signatures should be obtained from the student, parent, participating teachers, and participating Action Team members.

Functional Assessment Checklist
for Teachers and Staff (FACTS)

Student/Grade: _____   Date: _____

Interviewer: _____   Respondent(s): _____

Student profile: Please identify at least three strengths or contributions the student brings to school.

_____

_____

Problem Behavior(s): Identify problem behaviors

___ Tardy	___ Inapprop language	___ Disruptive	___ Theft
___ Unresponsive	___ Fight/physical aggress	___ Insubordination	___ Vandalism
___ Withdrawn	___ Verbal harassment	___ Work not done	___ Other_____

Describe problem behavior: _____

Identifying Routines: Where, when, and with whom problem behaviors are most likely.

Schedule (Times)	Activity	With Whom Does Problem Occur?	Likelihood of Problem Behavior	Specific Problem Behavior
			Low High 1 2 3 4 5 6	
			1 2 3 4 5 6	
			1 2 3 4 5 6	
			1 2 3 4 5 6	
			1 2 3 4 5 6	
			1 2 3 4 5 6	
			1 2 3 4 5 6	
			1 2 3 4 5 6	
			1 2 3 4 5 6	

Select 1–3 routines for further assessment. Select routines based on (1) similarity of activities (conditions) with ratings of 4, 5, or 6 and (2) similarity of problem behaviors(s). Complete the FACTS–Part B for each routine identified.

(continued)

FACTS–Part B

Student/Grade: _____ **Date:** _____

Interviewer: _____ **Respondent(s):** _____

Routine/Activities/Context: Which routine (only one) from the FACTS–Part A is assessed?

Routine/Activities/Context	Problem Behavior

Provide more detail about the problem behavior(s):

What does the problem behavior(s) look like?   **How often does the problem behavior(s) occur?**   **How long does the problem behavior(s) last when it does occur?**   **What is the intensity/level of danger of the problem behavior(s)?**

What are the events that predict when the problem behavior(s) will occur?

Related Issues (Setting Events)		Environmental Features	
___ illness	Other: ___	___ reprimand/correction	___ structured activity
___ drug use	_____	___ physical demands	___ unstructured time
___ negative social	_____	___ socially isolated	___ tasks too boring
___ conflict at home	_____	___ with peers	___ activity too long
___ academic failure	_____	___ other	___ tasks too difficult

What consequences are most likely to maintain the problem behavior(s)?

Things That Are Obtained		Things Avoided or Escaped From	
___ adult attention	Other: _____	___ hard tasks	Other: _____
___ peer attention	_____	___ reprimands	_____
___ preferred activity	_____	___ peer negatives	_____
___ money/things	_____	___ physical effort	_____

SUMMARY OF BEHAVIOR

Identify the summary that will be used to build a plan of behavior support

Setting Events and Predictors	Problem Behavior(s)	Maintaining Consequence(s)

How confident are you that the Summary of Behavior is accurate?

Not very confident					Very confident
1	2	3	4	5	6

(continued)

What current efforts have been used to control the problem behavior?

Strategies for Preventing Problem Behavior		Consequences for Problem Behavior	
___ schedule change	Other: _____	___ reprimand	Other: _____
___ seating change	_____	___ office referral	_____
___ curriculum change	_____	___ detention	_____

Instructions

The FACTS is a two-page interview used by school personnel who are building behavior support plans. The FACTS is intended to be an efficient strategy for initial functional behavioral assessment. The FACTS is completed by people (teachers, family, clinicians) who know the student best, and used to either build behavior support plans, or to guide more complete functional assessment efforts. The FACTS can be completed in a short period of time (5–15 min). Efficiency and effectiveness in completing the forms increases with practice.

How to Complete the FACTS–Part A

Step 1: Complete Demographic Information:

Indicate the name and grade of the student, the date the assessment data were collected, the name of the person completing the form (the interviewer), and the name(s) of the people providing information (respondents).

Step 2: Complete Student Profile

Begin each assessment with a review of the positive and contributing characteristics the student brings to school. Identify at least three strengths or contributions the student offers.

Step 3: Identify Problem Behaviors

Identify the specific student behaviors that are barriers to effective education, disrupt the education of others, interfere with social development, or compromise safety at school. Provide a brief description of exactly how the student engages in these behaviors. What makes his or her way of doing these behaviors unique? Identify the most problematic behaviors, but also identify any problem behaviors that occur regularly.

Step 4: Identify Where, When, and with Whom the Problem Behaviors Are Most Likely

A: List the times that define the student's daily schedule. Include times between classes, lunch, and before school, and adapt for complex schedule features (e.g., odd/even days) if appropriate.

B: For each time listed indicate the activity typically engaged in during that time (e.g., small-group instruction, math, independent art, transition).

C: Where appropriate indicate the people (adults and peers) with whom the student is interacting during each activity, and especially list the people the student interacts with when he or she engages in problem behavior.

D: Use the 1 to 6 scale to indicate (in general) which times/activities are most and least likely to be associated with problem behaviors. A "1" indicates low likelihood of problems, and a "6" indicates high likelihood of problem behaviors.

E: Indicate which problem behavior is *most likely* in any time/activity that is given a rating of 4, 5, or 6.

(continued)

Step 5: Select Routines for Further Assessment

Examine each time/activity listed as 4, 5, or 6 in the Table from Step 4. If activities are similar (e.g., activities that are unstructured; activities that involve high academic demands; activities with teacher reprimands; activities with peer taunting) and have similar problem behaviors, treat them as "routines for further analysis."

Select between one and three routines for further analysis. Write the name of the routine and the most common problem behavior(s). Within each routine identify the problem behavior(s) that are most likely or most problematic.

For *each* routine identified in Step 5 complete a FACTS–Part B

How to Complete the FACTS–Part B

Step 1: Complete Demographic Information

Identify the name and grade of the student, the date that the FACTS–Part B was completed, who completed the form, and who provided information for completing the form.

Step 2: Identify the Target Routine

List the targeted routine and problem behavior from the bottom of the FACTS–Part A. The FACTS–Part B provides information about *one* routine. Use multiple Part B forms if multiple routines are identified.

Step 3: Provide Specifics about the Problem Behavior(s)

Provide more detail about the features of the problem behavior(s). Focus specifically on the unique and distinguishing features, and the way the behavior(s) is disruptive or dangerous.

Step 4: Identify Events that Predict Occurrence of the Problem Behavior(s)

Within each routine what (a) setting events and (b) immediate preceding events predict when the problem behavior(s) will occur. What would you do to make the problem behaviors happen in this routine?

Step 5: Identify the Consequences that May Maintain the Problem Behavior

What consequences appear to reward the problem behavior? Consider that the student may get/obtain something he or she wants, or that he or she may escape/avoid something he or she finds unpleasant.

Identify the *most powerful* maintaining consequence with a "1," and other possible consequences with a "2" or "3." Do not check more than three options. The focus here is on the consequence that has the greatest impact.

When problems involve minor events that escalate into very difficult events, separate the consequences that maintain the minor problem behavior from the events that may maintain problem behavior later in the escalation.

Step 6: Define What Has Been Done to Date to Prevent/Control the Problem Behavior

In most cases, school personnel will have tried some strategies already. List events that have been tried, and organize these by (a) those things that have been done to prevent the problem from getting started, and (b) those things that were delivered as consequences to control or punish the problem behavior (or reward alternative behavior).

Step 7: Build a Summary Statement

The summary statement indicates the setting events, immediate predictors, problem behaviors, and maintaining consequences. The summary statement is the foundation for building an effective behavior support plan. Build the summary statement from the information in the FACTS–A and FACTS–B (especially the information in Steps 3, 4, and 5 of the FACTS–B). If you are confident that the summary statement is accurate enough to design a plan, move into plan development. If you are less confident, then continue the functional assessment by conducting direct observation.

Student-Guided Functional Assessment Interview (Primary)

Student: _____   Grade: _____   Sex: M F   IEP: Y N

Teacher: _____   School: _____

Interviewer: _____   Date: _____

OPENING

We are meeting today to find ways to change school, so that you like it more. This interview will take about 30 minutes. I can help you best if you answer honestly. You will not be asked anything that might get you in trouble.

STUDENT STRENGTHS AND SKILLS

1. What are things that you like to do, or do well, while at school? (e.g., activities, helping others).

2. What are classes/topics you do well in?

DEFINE THE BEHAVIORS OF CONCERN

Assist the student to identify specific behaviors that are resulting in problems in the school or classroom. Making suggestions or paraphrasing statements can help the student clarify her or his ideas.

What are the things you do that get you in trouble or are a problem? Prompts:-late to class?, talk out in class?, don't get work done?, fighting?

	Behavior	*Comment*
1.		
2.		
3.		
4.		
5.		
6.		
7.		

(continued)

Adapted from Reed, Thomas, Sprague, and Horner (1997). Copyright 1997 by Kluwer Academic/Plenum Publishing. Adapted by permission.

Which of the behaviors described are likely to occur together in some way? Do they occur about the same time? In some kind of predictable sequence or "chain"? In response to the same type of situation?

a.

b.

c.

Of those groups of behaviors which one is the most concern? The rest of the interview will focus on those behaviors.

a.

COMPLETE STUDENT SCHEDULE AND ROUTINE MATRIX

Assist the student to complete the schedule and routine matrices to show the routines and activities where they have difficulty with the behavior(s) they talked about. First have the student complete the schedule column (or have this column completed before the interview). Add any routines unique to the teacher's classroom.

We know that some times and activities are harder and easier for different people. Can you tell me which times during your day are easy and which are difficult? A "6" indicates it is likely that you will have a problem and a "1" indicates that no or few problem(s) occur. (Repeat for routines).

Student Schedule and Routine Matrix

Typical Schedule	Rating	Routines	Rating
	6 5 4 3 2 1	Getting help	6 5 4 3 2 1
	6 5 4 3 2 1	Getting material/drink, Sharpening pencil	6 5 4 3 2 1
	6 5 4 3 2 1	Working in groups	6 5 4 3 2 1
	6 5 4 3 2 1	Working independently (alone)	6 5 4 3 2 1
	6 5 4 3 2 1	Getting permission and Going to the restroom	6 5 4 3 2 1
	6 5 4 3 2 1	Transitions (between activities or locations)	6 5 4 3 2 1
	6 5 4 3 2 1	Working with substitute Teachers/volunteers	6 5 4 3 2 1
	6 5 4 3 2 1		6 5 4 3 2 1
	6 5 4 3 2 1		6 5 4 3 2 1

Assessing Activity Routines Form

Focus Individual _____

Date _____

Time	Routine/Activity	Likelihood of Problem Behavior	Type of Problem Behavior Most Likely
		Low High 1 2 3 4 5 6	
		1 2 3 4 5 6	
		1 2 3 4 5 6	
		1 2 3 4 5 6	
		1 2 3 4 5 6	
		1 2 3 4 5 6	
		1 2 3 4 5 6	
		1 2 3 4 5 6	
		1 2 3 4 5 6	
		1 2 3 4 5 6	
		1 2 3 4 5 6	
		1 2 3 4 5 6	
		1 2 3 4 5 6	
		1 2 3 4 5 6	
		1 2 3 4 5 6	
		1 2 3 4 5 6	
		1 2 3 4 5 6	
		1 2 3 4 5 6	
		1 2 3 4 5 6	

Brief Functional Assessment Interview Form

Student: _____ Date: _____

Behaviors of Concern:

Predictors:

Maintaining Function(s):

What Makes It Worse (Setting Events):

Summary Statement (Define by Routine)

Setting Event →	Predictor →	Problem Behavior →	Maintaining Function

Functional Behavioral Assessment Observation Form

Date __/__/__	Time __:__
Observer _____	
Student _____	
Classroom/School _____	

Setting Description:

Description of Behavior:

Time	Antecedents	Behaviors	Consequences

From Sugai and Colvin, *Effective School Consultation: An Interactive Approach* (1st ed.). © 1993. Adapted by permission of Brooks/Cole, an imprint of the Wadsworth Group, a division of Thomson Learning. Fax 800-730-2215.

Functional Assessment Observation Form

Name: _____

Starting Date: _____   Ending Date: _____

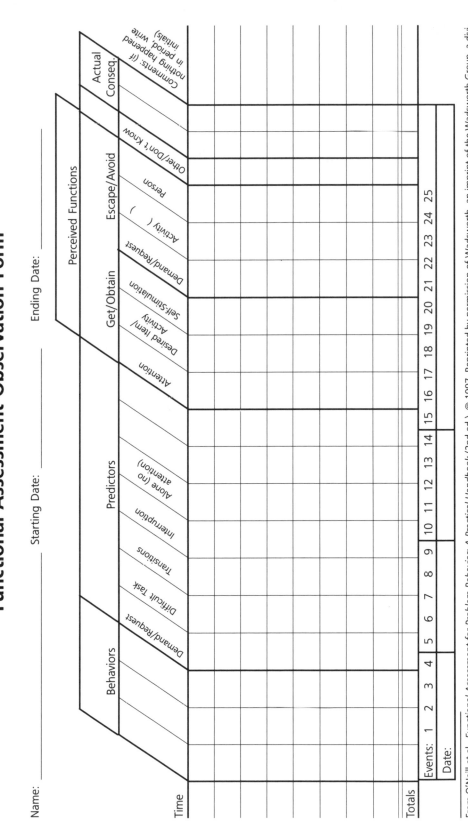

From O'Neill et al., *Functional Assessment for Problem Behavior: A Practical Handbook* (2nd ed.). © 1997. Reprinted by permission of Wadsworth, an imprint of the Wadsworth Group, a division of Thomson Learning. Fax 800-730-2215.

A Checklist for Assessing the Quality of Behavior Support Planning: Does the Plan (or Planning Process) Have These Features?

When developing and implementing behavior support plans, judge the degree to which each of the following has been considered:

G = Good   O = Okay   P = Poor   N = Not applicable

1. ____ Define academic and lifestyle *context* for behavior support
2. ____ Operational description of problem behaviors
3. ____ Problem *routines* identified
4. ____ Functional assessment hypotheses stated

5. Intervention/*Foundations* (issues that cut across routines)
   a) ____ health and physiology
   b) ____ communication
   c) ____ mobility
   d) ____ predictability
   e) ____ control/choice
   f) ____ social relationships
   g) ____ activity patterns

6. Intervention/*Prevention* (make problem behavior irrelevant)
   a) ____ schedule
   b) ____ curriculum
   c) ____ instructional procedures

7. Intervention/*Teaching* (make problem behavior inefficient)
   a) ____ replacement skills
   b) ____ new adaptive skills

8. Intervention/*Consequences*
   Extinction (make problem behavior ineffective)
   a) ____ minimize positive reinforcement
   b) ____ minimize negative reinforcement
   Reinforcement (make appropriate behavior more effective)
   a) ____ maximize positive reinforcement
   Punishment (if needed)
   a) ____ negative consequences contingent upon problem behavior
   Safety/Emergency Intervention Plan
   a) ____ clear plan for what to do if/when problem behaviors occur

(continued)

9. Evaluation and Assessment
   a) ____ define the information to be collected
   b) ____ define the measurement process
   c) ____ define decision-making process.

10. Ensure Contextual Fit
    a) ____ values
    b) ____ skills
    c) ____ resources
    d) ____ administrative system
    e) ____ perceptions that program is in best interest of student

References

Broussard, C. D., & Northrup, J. (1995). An approach to functional assessment and analysis of disruptive behavior in regular education classrooms. *School Psychology Quarterly, 10,* 151–164.

Carr, E. G. (1977). The motivation of self-injurious behavior: A review of some hypotheses. *Psychological Bulletin, 84,* 800–816.

Carr, E. G., Horner, R. H., Turnbull, A., Marquis, J., Magito-McLaughlin, D., McAtee, M., Smith, C. E., Anderson-Ryan, K. A., Ruef, M. B., & Doolabh, A. (1999). *Positive behavior support as an approach for dealing with problem behavior in people with developmental disabilities: A research synthesis.* Washington, DC: American Association on Mental Retardation.

Costenbader, V., & Markson, S. (1998). School suspension: A study with secondary school students. *Journal of School Psychology, 36,* 59–82.

Dunlap, G., White, R., Vera, A., Wilson, D., & Panacek, L. (1996). The effects of multicomponent, assessment-based curricular modifications on the classroom behavior of children with emotional and behavioral disorders. *Journal of Behavioral Education, 6*(4), 481–500.

DuPaul, G. J., & Ervin, R. A. (1996). Functional assessment of behavior related to ADHD: Linking assessment to intervention design. *Behavior Therapy, 27,* 601–622.

Dwyer, W. O., Leeming, F. C., Cobern, M. K., Porter, B. E., & Bryan, E. (1993). Critical review of behavioral interventions to preserve the environment: Research since 1980. *Environment and Behavior, 25,* 275–321.

Eccles, C., & Pitchford, M. (1997). Understanding and helping a boy with problems: A functional approach to behavior problems. *Educational Psychology in Practice, 13*(2), 115–121.

Ervin, R. A., DuPaul, G. J., Kern, L., & Friman, P. C. (1998). Classroom-based functional and adjunctive assessments: Proactive approaches to intervention selection for adolescents with Attention Deficit Hyperactivity Disorder. *Journal of Applied Behavior Analysis, 31,* 65–78.

Gable, R. (1999). Functional assessment in school settings. *Behavioral Disorders, 24*(2) 246–248.

Gresham, F. M., Gansle, K. A., Noell, G. H., Cohen, S., & Rosenblum, S. (1993). Treatment integrity of school-based behavioral intervention studies: 1980–1990. *School Psychology Review, 22,* 254–272.

Gresham, F. M., Quinn, M., & Restori, A. (1999). Methodological issues in functional analysis: Generalizability to other disability groups. *Behavioral Disorders, 24*(2), 180–182.

Gresham, F. M., Sugai, G., Horner, R. H., Quinn, M. M., & McInerney, M. (1998). *Classroom and school-wide practices that support children's social competence: A synthesis of research.* Washington, DC: American Institutes of Research and Office of Special Education Programs.

Horner, R. H., Sugai, G., & Todd, A. (1996). Comprehensive functional assessment in schools. Grant application submitted to the Office of Special Education, U.S. Department of Education. Eugene, OR: University of Oregon.

Horner, R. H., Sugai, G., Todd, A. W., & Lewis-Palmer, T. (1999–2000). Elements of behavior support plans: A technical brief. *Exceptionality, 8,* 205–216.

Individuals with Disabilities Education Act, Amendments of 1997. (1997). H.R. 5, 105th Congress, 1st Sess.

Iwata, B. A., Dorsey, M. F., Slifer, K. J., Bauman, K. E., & Richman, G. S. (1982). Toward a functional analysis of self-injury. *Analysis and Intervention in Developmental Disabilities, 2,* 3–20.

Leighton, M. S., O'Brien, E., Walking Eagle, K., Weiner, L., Wimberly, G., & Youngs, P. (1997). *Roles for education paraprofessionals in effective schools: An idea book.* Washington, DC: U.S. Department of Education.

Lewis, T. J., & Sugai, G. (1996). Functional assessment of problem behavior: A pilot investigation of the comparative and interactive effects of teacher and peer social attention on students in general education settings. *School Psychology Quarterly, 11,* 1–19.

Lewis, T. J., & Sugai, G. (1999). Effective Behavior Support: A Systems Approach to Proactive School-wide Management. *Focus on Exceptional Children, 31*(6), 1–24.

Loeber, R., & Farrington, D. (1998). *Serious and violent juvenile offenders: Risk factors and successful interventions.* London: Sage.

Luiselli, J. K., & Cameron, M. J. (Eds.). (1998). *Antecedent control: Innovative approaches to behavioral support.* Baltimore: Brookes.

March, R., Horner, R. H., Lewis-Palmer, L., Brown, D., Crone, D., Todd, A. W., & Carr, E. (2000). *Functional Assessment Checklist for Teachers and Staff (FACTS).* Eugene: Department of Educational and Community Supports, University of Oregon.

Mayer, G. R. (1995). Preventing antisocial behavior in the schools. *Journal of Applied Behavior Analysis, 28,* 467–478.

National Education Goals Report. (1995). *http://inet.ed.gov/pubs/goals/.*

Nelson, J. R., Roberts, M., Mathur, S., & Rutherford, R. B. (1999). Has public policy exceeded our knowledge base? A review of the functional assessment literature. *Behavioral Disorders, 24,* 169–179.

Nippe, G. E., Lewis-Palmer, T., & Sprague, J. (1998). *The student-directed functional assessment: An analysis of congruence between student self-report and direct obser-*

vation. Manuscript submitted for publication. Department of Education and Community Supports, University of Oregon, Eugene.

O'Neill, R. E., Horner, R. H., Albin, R. W., Sprague, J. R., Storey, K., & Newton, J. S. (1997). *Functional assessment for problem behavior: A practical handbook* (2nd ed.). Pacific Grove, CA: Brooks/Cole.

Reed, H. K., Thomas, E. S., Sprague, J. R., & Horner, R. H. (1997). The student guided functional assessment interview: An analysis of student and teacher agreement. *Journal of Behavioral Education, 7*, 33–49.

Royer, E. (1995). Behaviour disorders, exclusion and social skills: Punishment is not education. *Therapeutic Care and Education, 4*, 32–36.

Schmidt, W., & Finnegan, J. (1993). *The race without a finish line*. San Francisco: Jossey-Bass.

Sugai, G., Bullis, M., & Cumblad, C. (1997). Skill development and support of educational personnel. *Journal of Emotional and Behavioral Disorders, 5*, 55–64.

Sugai, G., Horner, R. H., Dunlap, G., Hieneman, M., Lewis, T. J., Nelson, C. M., Scott, T., Liaupsin, C., Sailor, W., Turnbull, A. P., Turnbull, H. R., III, Wickam, D., Ruef, M., & Wilcox, B. (2000). Applying positive behavioral support and functional behavioral assessment in schools. *Journal of Positive Behavioral Interventions, 2*, 131–143.

Sugai, G., Sprague, J. R., Horner, R. H., & Walker, H. M. (2000). Preventing school violence. The use of office discipline referrals to assess and monitor school-wide discipline interventions. *Journal of Emotional and Behavioral Disorders, 8*(2), 94–101.

Taylor-Greene, S., Brown, D., Nelson, L., Longton, J., Gassman, T., Cohen, J., Swartz, J., Horner, R. H., Sugai, G., & Hall, S. (1997). School-wide behavioral support: Starting the year off right. *Journal of Behavioral Education, 7*(1), 99–112.

Todd, A. W., Horner, R. H., Sugai, G., & Colvin, G. (1999). Individualizing school-wide discipline for students with chronic problem behaviors: A team approach. *Effective School Practices, 17*, 72–82.

Turnbull, R., Rainbolt, K., & Buchele-Ash, A. (1997). *Individuals with Disabilities Education Act: Digest and significance of 1997 amendments*. Beach Center on Families and Disability, Lawrence, KS: University of Kansas.

Vollmer, T. R., & Northrup, J. (1996). Some implications of functional analysis for school psychology. *School Psychology Quarterly, 11*, 76–92.

Walker, H., Colvin, G., & Ramsey, E. (1995). *Antisocial behavior in public schools: Strategies and best practices*. Pacific Grove, CA: Brooks/Cole.

Walker, H., Horner, R., Sugai, G., Bullis, M., Sprague, J., Bricker, D., & Kaufman, M. (1996). Integrated approaches to preventing antisocial behavior patterns among school-aged youth. *Journal of Emotional and Behavior Disorders, 4* (4), 194–209.

Wilcox, B. L., Turnbull, H. R., & Turnbull, A. P. (1999–2000). Behavioral issues and IDEA: PBS and the FBA in the disciplinary context. *Exceptionalities, 8*(3), 173–187.

Index

Action Team
  agenda for, 98f
  functions of, 88–91, 103, 105–106
  membership of, 102–103
  Partnership Agreement for, 103, 104f
Activity routines, form for assessing, 153
Agendas, content of, 97, 98f, 99f
Antecedents of problem behavior, 13, 62
  description of, 138–139
  summary of, 130, 132, 139

B

Behavior
  appropriate
    documenting in BSP, 63, 64f–66f, 67
    increasing, 13
    teaching, 35
  assessing changes in, 72–76
    with behavior rating scale, 73, 74f, 75, 75f
    with frequency count, 72, 73f
    with observations, 76, 76f
  functionality of, 11–12, 140
  inappropriate, function of, 12
  predictability of, 12–13
  problem. See Problem behavior
Behavior management, resources for, 9
Behavior problems. See Problem behavior
Behavior rating scale, 73, 74f, 75, 75f
Behavior support plans, 4
  checklist for assessing, 69f
  design of, 55–69
    competing behaviors in, 55–56, 57f–59f, 60
    contextual fit of, 60–62
    individualizing, 62–63
  designing, 43–44
  documenting, 63, 64f–66f, 67–68, 67t
  evaluating/modifying, 70–84
    for changes in behavior, 71–73, 74f, 75, 75f
    data-based decision in, 82–84
    documentation of, 76, 77f–79f, 80
    for feasibility/fidelity, 80–81
    maintenance plan based on, 84
    observations in, 76, 76f
    for parent, teacher, student satisfaction, 80–81
    rationale for, 70–71
  flow chart of, 26f

Behavior support plans *(cont.)*
  and functional nature of behavior,
      11–12
  home-school note for, 61
  implementation of, assessing
      feasibility/fidelity of, 80–81
  parent, teacher, student satisfaction
      with, 81
  protocol for, 129–145
    instructions for completing, 137–
      145
  quality of, checklist for assessing,
      163–164
  references on, 68
  reinforcers in, 63
  steps in, 24–26, 25t
  tools for developing, 9
Behavior support systems, continuum
      of, 114–115
Behavior support team
  Action Team of, 88–91
  collaboration among, 96–109
    procedure for, 100, 101f, 102–103,
      104f, 105–106
    structure for, 96–1097, 98f, 99–
      100, 99f
  core team of, 88–95
  follow-up survey for, 107f–109f
  member roles and responsibilities,
      90f, 93–95
  membership of, 91–93
  references for, 122–124
  referral to, 30. See also Referrals
  structure of, 88–91, 89f
  training outcomes for, 115–116
Behavioral assessment, functional. See
      Functional behavioral assessment
Behavioral interventions, 24–26
  effective, 4
    support for, 34
  planning, 4
  resources for, 9–10
  selecting, 135, 143–144
Behavioral systems, 15f
Behaviors, competing, 55–56, 57f–59f, 60
BSPs. See Behavior support plans

C

Check-in/Check-out system, 18–19
Competing Behavior Pathway
  building, 134, 142–143
  form for, 80
  steps in, 55–56, 57f–59f, 60
Consequences
  description of, 130, 132, 139
  identifying, 15
  rewarding, 13
Contextual fit, 60–62
Crisis intervention
  BSP for, 67–68, 67t
  plans for, 10

D

Decisions, data-based, 82–84
Disabilities. See also Individuals with
      Disabilities Education Act
  behavior problems of children with,
      IEP suggestions for, 5
Discipline
  lack of, 3
  references on, 122–124
  student referrals for, 16, 17t. See also
      Referrals
Divorce, FBA implications of, 44

E

Evaluation plans
  designing, 144–145
  documenting, 76, 77f–79f, 80
  form for, 136

F

Families. See also Parents
  interviews of, 44, 45f–46f, 47
FBA. See Functional behavioral
      assessment
Federal government, FBA requirements
      of, 4–5
Feedback, for student, 73, 75

Frequency counts, 72, 73f
Functional analysis, 24
  references on, 54
Functional Assessment Checklist, 35
  form for, 147–150
Functional assessment interviews. See
  Interviews
Functional behavioral assessment
  case examples of, 29–30
  changing applications of, 7
  components of, 15–24, 15f
  conducting, 29–54
  and continuum of behavior support
    systems, 114–115
  current context for, 3–10
  decision rules for, 20, 21f
  federal requirements for, 4–5
  flow chart of, 26f
  full, 19f, 20, 22t, 23, 44–53
    interviews in, 44, 45f–46f, 47, 48f–
      49f, 50
    observation in, 50–51, 52f, 53, 53f
    functional analysis in, 22t, 24
      references on, 54
  generating within-building support
    for. See Schools, building FBA
    support in
  hypothesis statement in, 22–23
  IDEA requirements and, 20, 110–
    111
  legislative demands for, 5–6
  maturing technology for, 7
  model for, 15–16, 15f, 18
  parent, teacher, student satisfaction
    with, 81
  procedural efficiency of, 7–8
  protocol for, 129–145
    instructions for completing, 137–
      145
  requests for assistance forms in, 30,
    31f–33f, 34–35
  requirements and commitments for,
    111–115
  resources for, 6–9, 112–114
    financial, 114
    time, 112–114, 113t

simple, 18–19, 19f, 21–23, 22t, 35–44
  teacher interview in, 35, 36f–41f,
    42
  testable hypothesis in, 43–44
  steps in, 21
Functional Behavioral Assessment-
  Behavior Support Plan Protocol,
  35

H

Home-school notes, 61
Human behavior. See Behavior
Hunger, as factor in problem behavior,
  13–14
Hypotheses, testable, 130, 132, 133,
  141–142
  confirming/modifying, 142
  creating, 140
  developing, 43–44
  testing, 53

I

IDEA. See Individuals with Disabilities
  Education Act
IEP. See Individualized Education Plan
  team
Individualized Education Plan team, 5
Individuals with Disabilities Education
  Act
  amendments to, 5
  FBA provisions of, 110–111
  requirements of, objectives for
    meeting, 110
  and three-tiered model of FBA, 20
Ineffectiveness, of problem behavior,
  14–15
Inefficiency, of problem behavior, 14
Interventions. See Behavioral
  interventions
Interviews
  brief, form for, 155
  ending, 140
  FBA, tools for, 8–9
  instructions for, 137

Interviews *(cont.)*
  of parents/families, 44, 45f–46f, 47
  student-guided, form for, 151–152
  of students, 47, 48f–49f, 50, 131–136,
      141
  of teachers, 35, 36f–41f, 42
  with teacher/staff/parents, 129

L

Leadership models, 120–122
Legislation, on FBA, 5–6

M

Maintenance plans, 84
Meetings
  attendance at, 99–100
  efficient, 97, 99–100

N

Note taking, 100
  form for, 101f

O

Observations
  for assessing behavioral change, 76, 76f
  conducting, 142
  forms for, 157, 159
  guidelines and purposes, 50–51, 52f,
      53, 53f
  tools for, 9

P

Paperclip transfer strategy, 72
Parents
  on behavior support team, 93
  follow-up survey of, 107f
  interviews of, 44, 45f–46f, 47, 129
  reaction of, to FBA-BSP process, 81
Partnership Agreement, 103, 104f
Principal, behavior support team roles
      of, 91–92

Problem behavior
  assessment/intervention for,
      changing thinking about, 11–
      26
  case studies in, 29–53
  categories of, 114
  changeable nature of, 13–15
  of children with disabilities, IEP
      suggestions for, 5
  description of, 131, 138
  efficiency factor in, 12
  environmental versus pathological
      causes of, 13
  functions of, 140
  at individual student system level,
      18
  making ineffective, 14–15
  making inefficient, 14
  making irrelevant, 13–14
  operational definitions of, 34–35
  predictors/antecedents of, 13, 62
  problems associated with, 3–4
  proportion of student body referred
      for, 16, 17t
  reducing and replacing, 55–56, 57f–
      59f, 60
  reinforcing consequences of, 4, 15
  student identification of, 47, 50
  teaching replacements for, 14
  triggers of, 4
Punishment, ineffectiveness of, 4, 30,
      34

R

Referrals
  in assessment process, 30
  forms for, 100, 102
  for individual student system level
      behavior, 18
  proportion of student body receiving,
      16, 17t
Reinforcers, 63
Request for Assistance, forms for, 30,
      31f–33f, 34–35, 100, 102, 127–
      128

S

Schools
  behavioral systems in, 15–16, 15f,
    18
  building FBA support in, 4, 110–
    124
    leadership models for, 120–122
    model for, 115–119
  changing job description of, 111–
    112
School-Wide Information System, 16
Students
  behavioral categories of, 114
  feedback for, 73, 75
  follow-up survey of, 108f

interviewing, 47, 48f–49f, 50, 129,
    131–136, 141
  reaction of, to FBA-BSP process, 81
SWIS. See School-Wide Information System
Systems, FBA and, 15–16, 15f, 18

T

Teachers
  follow-up survey of, 109f
  interviews of, 35, 36f–41f, 42, 129
  reaction of, to FBA-BSP process, 81
Timekeeper, role of, 99
Training, for behavior support team,
    115–119, 119f